Acknowledgements

I wrote my first textbook on Dental Photography with a colleague, Dr Phil Wander, in 1987. In 1998, I left practice to work for what was then "The Dental Reference Service" until the "Care Quality Commission (CQC)" took over that role in 2011. It is obvious from the above dates that when I was commissioned to write a book on "Dental Photography", I had no direct access to patients or surgeries.

I am lost for words as to how to thank my younger colleagues for their support both with allowing access to surgeries, modeling, taking images, etc. I am equally grateful to three of my grandchildren, Abbie and Sammy Hass, and Jamie Simon who ran the risk of being placed in front of a camera every time they paid a visit.

Acknowledgment of images are given in the text as they arise and if not individually acknowledged, the images will have been taken by the author.

Four colleagues deserve special mention, Dr Mahul Patel who photographed Dr Diana Bennett and Dr Neel Jaiswal who photographed his wife Dr Kamal Mistry.

Further thanks are due to Dr Souphiyeh Samizadeh and Dr Alexandra Day for their help with facial esthetics.

Thanks are due to Tony Knight of Knight Dental Design for access to his "studio" and generous loan of models and to Bryan Matthews of "Tusk Dental Laboratories" for both loan of models and images.

Further thanks are due to Olympus UK for the loan of a camera and flash system and Canon UK for the loan of the M50 mirrorless body 250D and 800D DSLR.

Thanks to the Royal Free Trust and Barts Trust for their hospital protocol on the use of mobile phones. I am very grateful to Dr Aws Alani BDS, MFDS MSc FDSRCS for access to his LLM Thesis submitted in 2017 to Cardiff University entitled, "Digital Media and the Dental Patient: A legal perspective". Last but by no means least, my sincere thanks to Harsha Madan, and her team at JP Medical Publishers for all the hard work and support from the beginning. Literally as the last i was dotted and t's crossed on the final proof, Harsha left on maternity leave, I send my congratulations on the safe arrival of her son and wish her and family well for the future.

Contacts and further reading

Dental Photography: Wander and Gordon BDJ 1987
Digital Dental Photography " A clinicians guide:" Steve Ratcliff DDS
Dental Photography: Krzysztof Chmielewski: Quintessence Publishing
Smile Design A Patient's Guide Dr Elliot Mechanic BSc DDS EC Dental Solutions Inc
Smile Transformations: Knight Dental Design
Guidelines on Social Media: General Dental Council
Information Commissioner's Office, BYOD (Bring Your Own Device)
"Riskwise" Dental Protection Issue 17 January 2018. "The Device in your pocket" Dr Philip Johnstone.
Aesthetic & Restorative Dentistry: Material Selection & Technique Douglas A Terry and Willi Geller
Esthetic Dentistry A Patient's Guide Dr Elliot Mechanic BSc DDS
Photographic Documentation & Evaluation in Cosmetic Dentistry American Academy of Cosmetic Dentistry
Microscopic Dentistry A Practical Guide by Carl Zeiss is recommended.

www.canon.co.uk
www.nikon.co.uk
www.olympus.co.uk
www.intro2020.co.uk For Metz products
www.kenro.co.uk For Kenro and Nissin products
www.lumiquest.com For Lumiquest boxes and bouncers
organicdentistry.store@gmail.com For LDB bouncers
www.photomed.net For Photomed products
www.dinecorp.com For Lester Dine products
www.agnos.com For Agnos products
www.owlbracket.com For Owl brackets
www.emulation.me For Axis brackets and Polar_eyes
www.dentalize.eu For polarising systems
www.sigma-imaging-uk.com For Sigma products
www.doctorseyes.com For Doctorseyes products
ramezani@t-online.de For Sara Led products
www.dentalphotomaster.com For Molinaris bracket and other accessories
www.jakobi-dental.com For Jakobi products
www.adaptalux.com For Adaptalux products
www.imi.org.uk For IMI National Guidelines Consent to Clinical Photography (Institute of Medical Illustrators)
www.forensicssource.com For forensic rulers
www.imi.org.uk Institute of Medical Illustrators for information and guidance on clinical photography
www.rotolight.com For Rotolight
www.tamron.co.uk For Tamron
info@denscreen.co.uk For Covid advice
sales@henryschein.co.uk For Covid advice

Dental photography and COVID-19

The current pandemic has thrown routine medical and dental treatment into turmoil, and those involved in the 1980s will remember how HIV affected practice protocol. With hindsight the "nuisance" at the time of wearing gloves and masks seems almost laughable today.

This book was finalised through the current COVID-19 pandemic which gave rise to the following considerations.

Using DSLR cameras

Most dental photography occurs in routine practice. These cameras and accessories cannot be sterilised and the current protocol if the operator is using the camera, is to remove gloves, use camera, wash hands and re-glove.

Routine practice with DSLR

Before any routine practice is carried out, it is assumed that some form of triage has been undertaken. Only after risk assessing each patient individually, treatment can be carried out in a reasonably normal manner. In the UK "DenScreen" offers training courses, triage tools and testing equipment to help dentistry get back to routine practice. Their antibody pin-prick test is 99% accurate, giving a result in 10 minutes. The results of the triage and test add empirical evidence to enhance risk assessments, enabling practices to resume routine dentistry. Henry Schein also offer COVID-19 advice.

In this environment, the camera can safely be used as earlier. One can stretch cling film tightly over a standard ring flash and lens without reducing image quality. Probably this will give the patient a greater sense of security rather than being a necessary precaution (**Figure 1**).

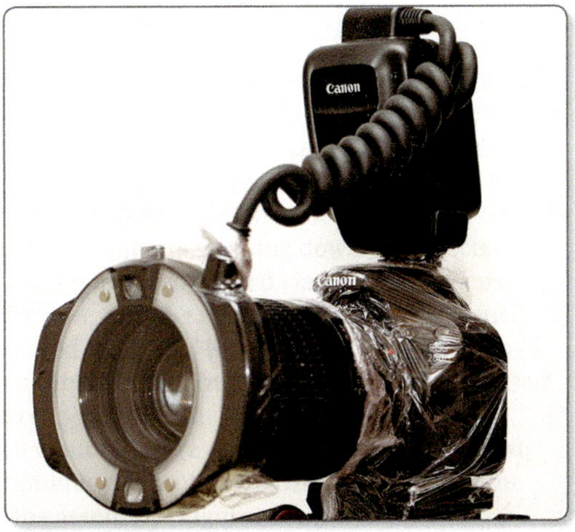

Figure 1 Camera with cling film over flash and separately over the body.

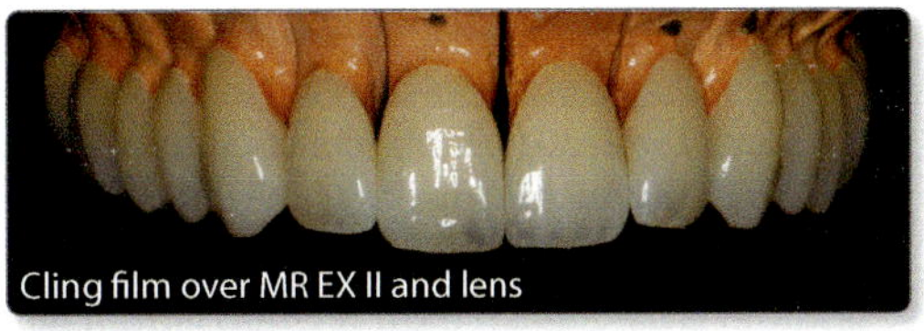

Figure 2a With cling film.

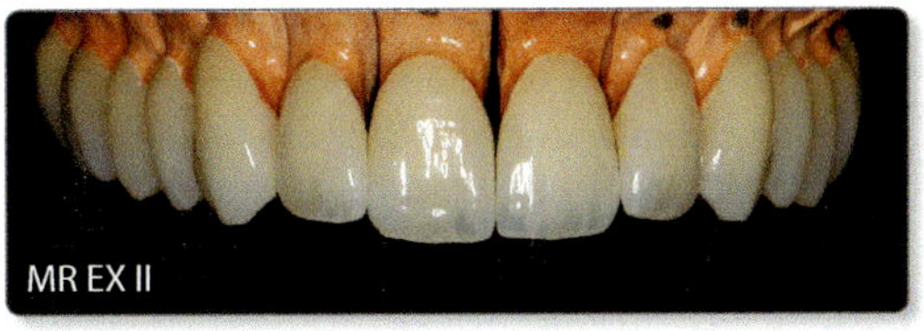

Figure 2b Without cling film.

Figures 2a and **b** show that the film has no deleterious effect on the image. The text describes a method of setting up the camera so that it and flash just need turning "on" and the only physical change required is setting the field of view.

If a camera system that can be disinfected is required, there are three systems described in Chapter 5 that would fulfil these criteria.

The author wishes to point out that he has no financial interest in any product mentioned in the text.

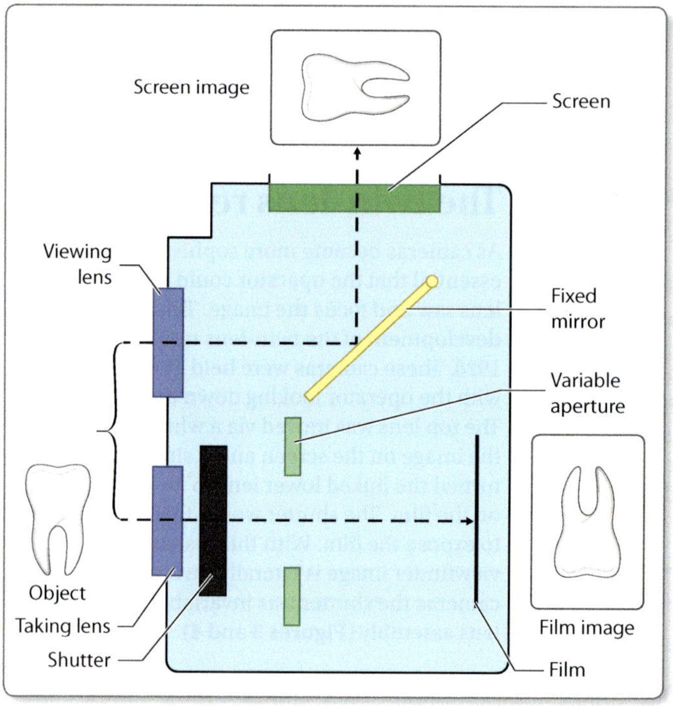

Figure 3 Twin-lens reflex camera.

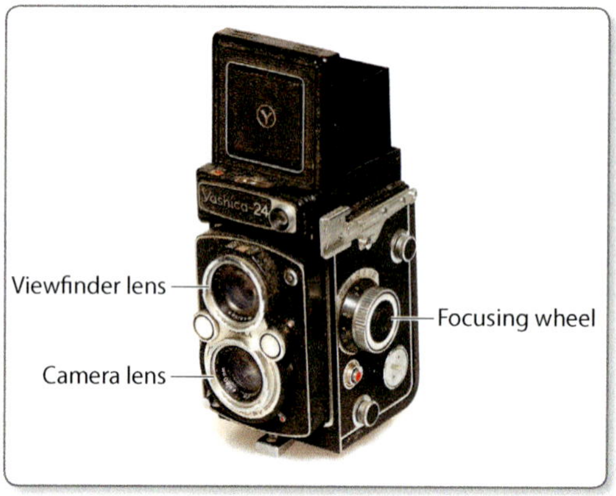

Figure 4 Yashica twin-lens reflex c 1950.
(*Courtesy:* Dr Peter Gordon)

The 35 mm single-lens reflex

The 35 mm SLR first produced in 1948, follows the same principle as above but on a smaller scale. In addition, the image from the mirror is diverted via a pentaprism to the eye enabling the user to see exactly what the lens is 'seeing.' The prism renders the eye level image both laterally correct and the right way up! Current DSLR cameras follow the same optical principals with a sensor now replacing film. In these cameras, the shutter is no longer part of the lens assembly, but a curtain system is placed directly in front of the film/sensor and referred to as a 'focal plane shutter' (**Figure 6**). The operation of a DSLR is fully described in Chapter 1.

Single-lens reflex cameras have been the mainstay of dental photography for over 60 years. They use 35 mm film in a cassette (see **Figure 7**) producing images in a 36 × 24 mm format, either in colour as the transparency **(Figure 8)** or as a negative for monochrome or colour prints.

The 35 mm cameras were developed in two directions, the SLR as described above, and the 'Rangefinder' models which were much smaller and represented by the compact cameras today (**Figure 9**).

The essential difference between the two types of camera being the lens of the SLR was part of the viewfinder system, the rangefinder cameras incorporated a 'telescope' type viewfinder

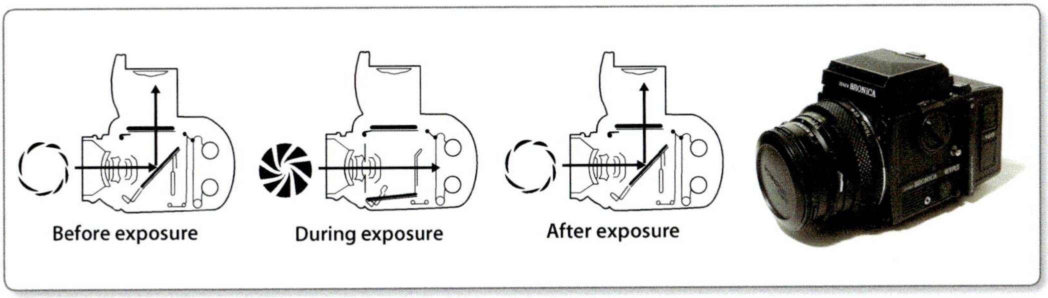

Figure 5 Single-lens reflex camera 6 × 6 cm format.
(*Courtesy:* Alex Falk of 'Mr Cad')

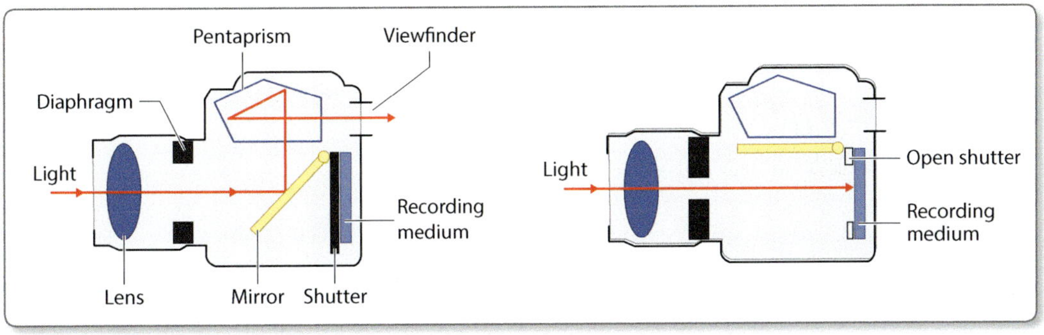

Figure 6 35 mm single-lens reflex camera.

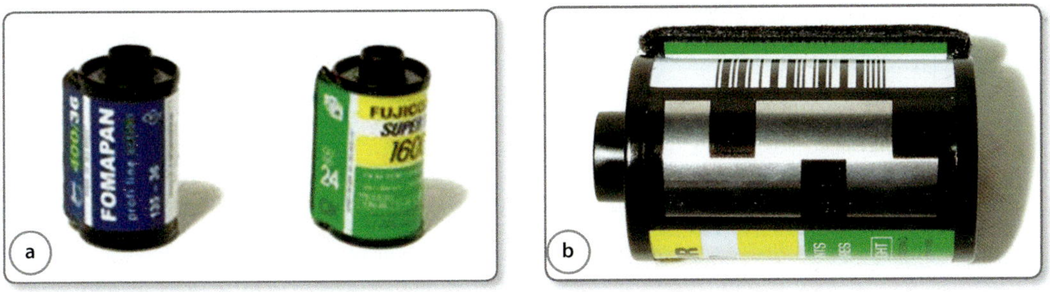

Figure 7 (a) 35 mm film cassettes. (b) Cassette shows DX coding which automatically sets the ISO in 35 mm cameras after 1985.
(*Courtesy:* Alex Falk of 'Mr Cad')

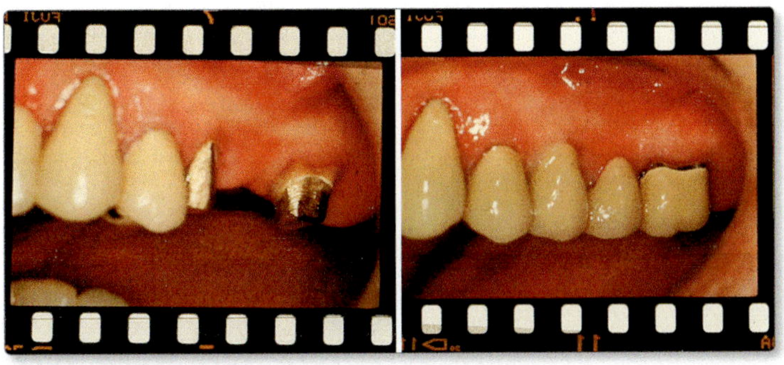

Figure 8 Before and after images taken on 35 mm slide film showing consistency of image size and position.
(*Courtesy:* Dr Peter Gordon)

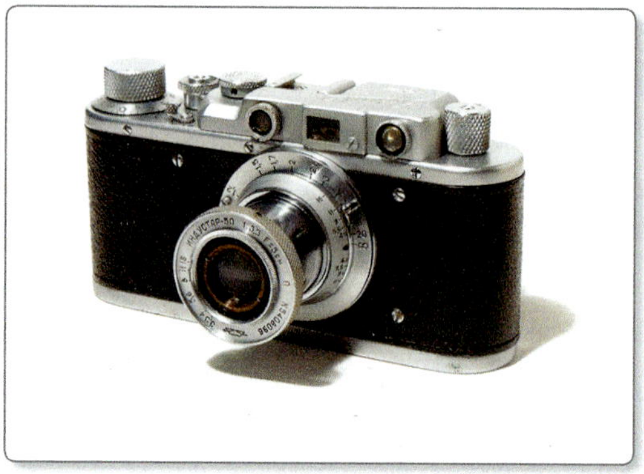

Figure 9 35 mm rangefinder camera.
(*Courtesy*: Alex Falk of 'Mr Cad')

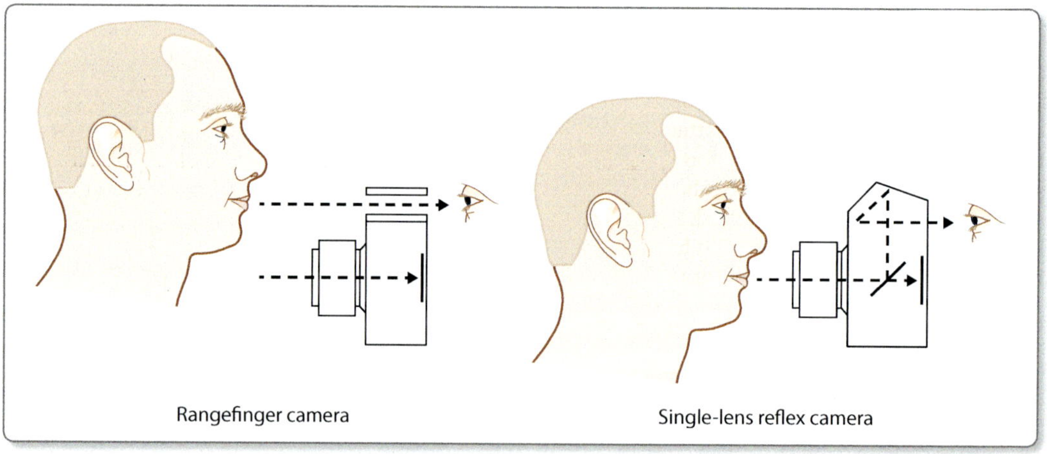

Figure 10 Parallax (a) Rangefinder camera, (b) Single-lens reflex camera.

showing a similar view to the lens. When interchangeable lenses were developed for these cameras, separate camera-mounted viewfinders were required. One further complication and important in the field of close-up photography is the problem of parallax.

From **Figure 10**, it is obvious that the closer the rangefinder camera is to the subject, the greater the difference between what the lens captures and what the viewfinder 'sees.' With the reflex camera the viewfinder shows exactly what the lens 'sees.'

1 The DSLR body

Introduction

The current digital single-lens reflex (DSLR) camera **Figure 1** is still the benchmark standard for this genre of photography and its function will be described in detail. Other available systems will be mentioned separately.

Camera function

Light from the subject passes through the aperture ring onto a mirror, reflected to and focused on a matte screen and then directed to the viewfinder/eye via a prism. When the shutter is operated, the mirror flips out of view, the shutter exposes the sensor for the appropriate period and the mirror returns to its original position, the cycle completing in a fraction of a second. Suffice to say in 'viewfinder' mode the aperture is fully open and closes electronically to the pre determined setting when the shutter is operated. As the shutter is placed directly in front of the sensor, it is known as a focal plane shutter. Control of exposure will be discussed fully later in the book.

Single-lens reflex cameras were initially designed to be held and used at eye level. With most current digital cameras, the rear screen can also be used as the viewfinder; however, dental systems can be both heavy and bulky, so for reasons of stability, eye level viewing is recommended.

The DSLR is based on the identical principle of the earlier cameras with a sensor replacing film. The major difference in practical terms is whilst the film is moved for sequential images, the sensor is fixed, and the 'images' are transferred electronically in milliseconds to a capture card, usually an SD card. These cards incorporate a slider to protect images from inadvertent deletion (**Figure 2**).

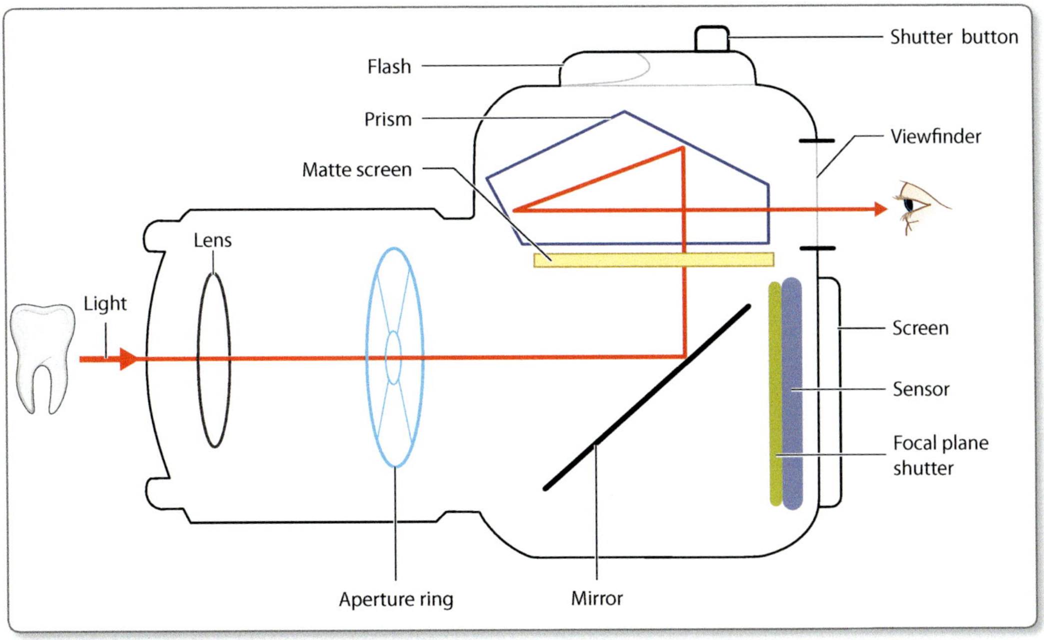

Figure 1 Diagram of digital single-lens reflex (DSLR) camera.

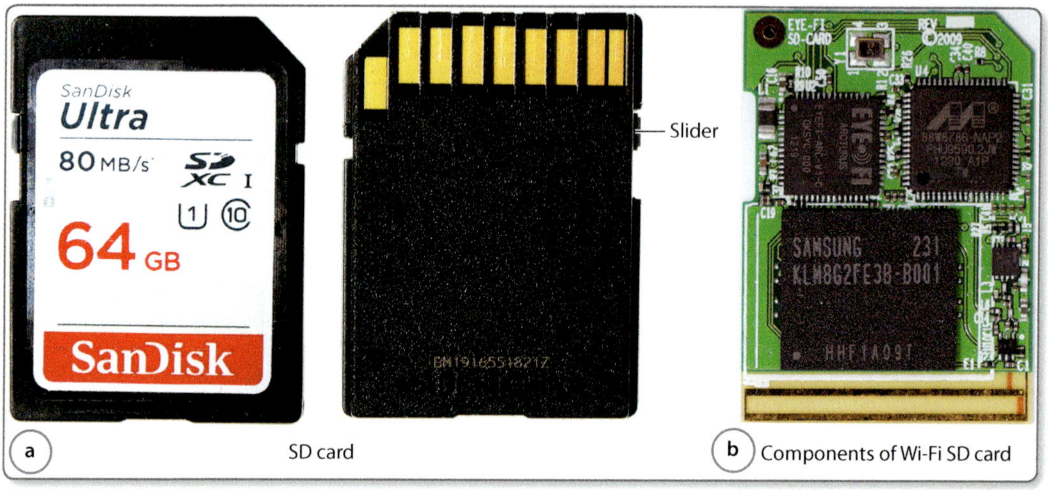

Figure 2 (a) SD card; (b) Components of Wi-Fi SD card.

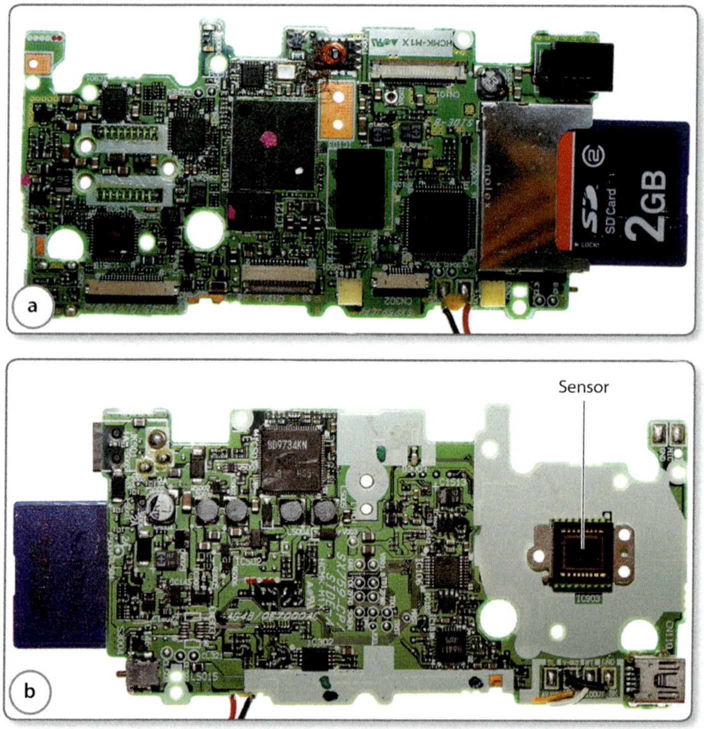

Figures 3a and b Components of a compact digital camera.

The image on a digital camera is captured by light sensitive pixels (picture elements) on the sensor with upwards of 15 million being the norm. The process of producing an image is complex, (see **Figure 3**), and outside the remit of this text. Each pixel will represent one dot of the original subject and theoretically the more pixels on a sensor the higher the quality of the image, however there can be a tradeoff. Take the sensor (**Figure 3b**), to accommodate 20 million pixels, each one would be smaller than the same size sensor with 15 million pixels, the larger pixels can sometimes give a better result than the smaller, so it is not always a case of more is better.

Current DSLR cameras can be divided into two groups, those incorporating a full frame or 24 × 36 mm sensor and the most popular using a smaller 'cropped' sensor. Canon APS-C sensors are 22.4 × 14.8 mm and the Nikon slightly larger at 24 × 16 mm. All the current lenses have been developed from those designed for 35 mm film cameras and their specifications in terms of focal length, maximum aperture and magnification ratios on macro lenses still relate to that format. Most cameras used in dental photography today will have cropped sensors rendering the details on magnification ratios inaccurate and they will be addressed where appropriate (**Figure 4**).

Components of a DSLR system

A DSLR camera body is the basis of a photographic system with the operator choosing the appropriate lens and other accessories for specific applications.

A basic camera system will consist of a camera body, a lens, and all but some top end 'professional' cameras, will incorporate a built-in flash unit.

A camera system for dental photography will require a body, appropriate macro lens, and usually a flash illumination system which are described in detail later. From the dental photography point of view 'entry level' camera bodies are totally suitable.

Focusing

Focusing can be achieved automatically or manually by adjusting the focus ring on the lens. Either way, using the camera at eye level the image will be seen on the focusing screen. Typically, this is ground glass with etched markings to facilitate alignment of the subject (**Figure 5**).

Dioptre wheel

If the operator looks into the viewfinder whilst aiming the camera at a white ceiling or similar, he/she can adjust the sharpness of the etchings by turning the 'dioptre' wheel situated near the viewfinder. This will adjust the viewfinder's optical system to the user's individual eyesight (**Figure 6**).

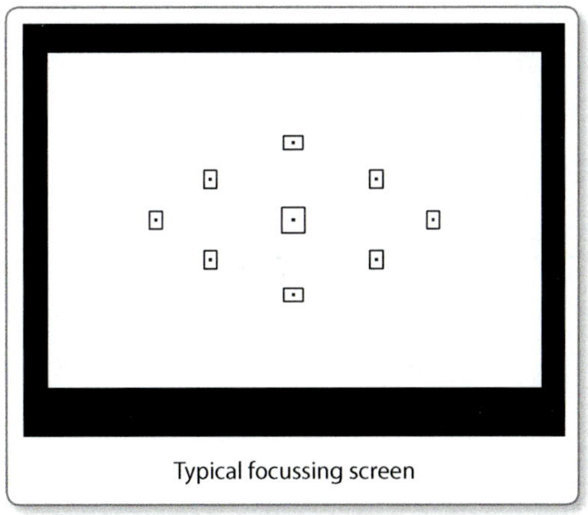

Figure 5 Typical focussing screen.

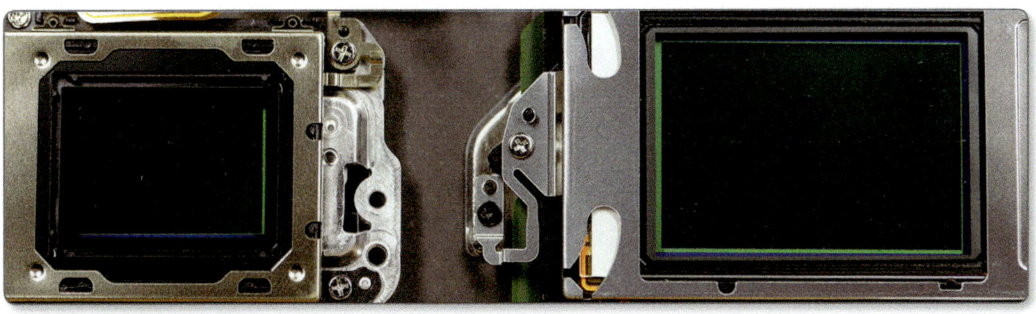

Figure 4 Direct comparison of Canon cropped and full frame sensors. (*Courtesy:* Canon sensors loaned courtesy of Mick Edwards FIXATION Ltd.)

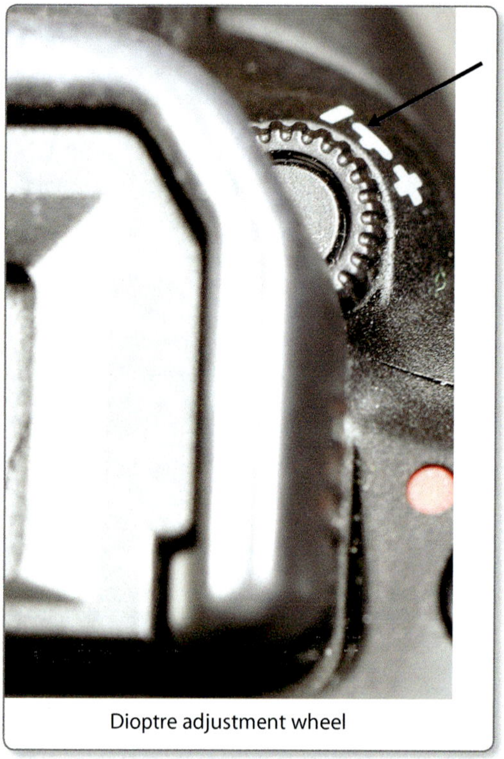

Figure 6 Dioptre adjustment wheel.

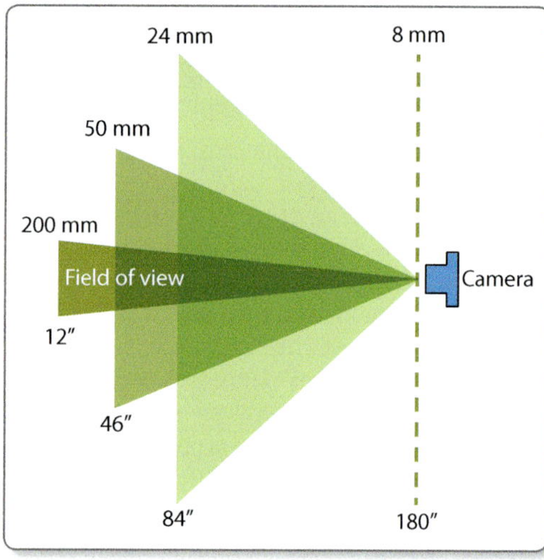

Figure 7 Fields of view at various focal lengths.

The lens

Focal length determines the angle of the field of view, the lower the focal length number, the wider the field of view (**Figure 7**).

When close-up photography is considered, the focal length is critical as it also controls the lens to subject distance (working distance) and perspective.

On a cropped sensor camera, a 35 mm lens covers what the eye sees and on a full frame system a 50 mm lens would be the standard.

Lenses can be divided into two groups, those with a fixed focal length and therefore a fixed field of view, are known as PRIME lenses. The other group and very popular for general photography have a variable field of view, e.g. 24–200 mm and are known as ZOOM lenses.

Specialist lenses for close-up photography, macro lenses, are a subgroup of PRIME lenses and are available in a variety of fixed focal lengths.

The advantage of a DSLR system is the ability to purchase the body individually and choose an appropriate lens for a given situation.

Apart from the optics, lenses contain one major physical component, the aperture or diaphragm. This is a variable-sized opening controlled electronically from the camera body (see **Figure 10**).

Exposure

Ambient light exposure

Exposure is determined by the intensity of light hitting the sensor, and the duration. Three factors control this: The size of the lens aperture, designated by ‘f’ numbers, which control the amount of light hitting the sensor; the shutter speed, which controls the duration of exposure; and the sensitivity of the sensor to light, which is determined by the ISO setting. They are interrelated; a change in one factor will require a change in one or both of the others (**Figure 8**).

Consider **Figure 9**, the ISO has been set at 800. Note that the exposure times differ by one half from left to right and get longer, and that the sizes of holes get smaller from left to right. Although the aperture numbers designated ‘f’ appear unrelated, each hole from left to right is exactly twice the area of its predecessor. Thus, in every combination above, the amount of light passing through each aperture and reaching the sensor, is the same. Should the sensitivity be halved, i.e. ISO 400, correct exposure would be achieved by moving the shutter speeds one place to the left and the exposure time at f22 would be 1/7.5 seconds (i.e. doubling the exposure) (**Figure 9**).

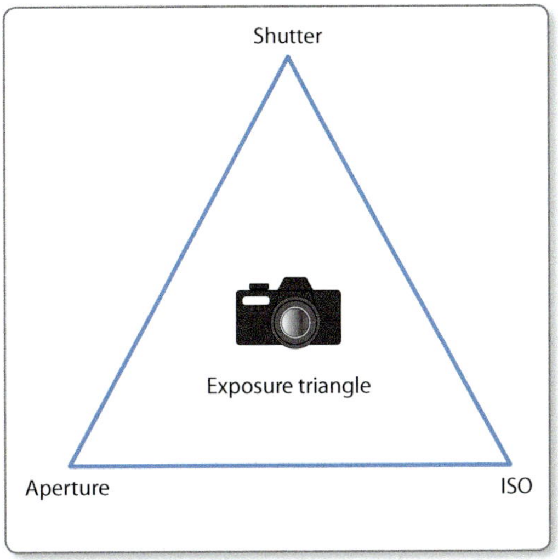

Figure 8 Exposure triangle.

The aperture size is of prime importance in close-up/dental photography as it controls 'depth of field' (DoF) which will be discussed in detail in a later chapter. **Figure 11** taken with apertures of f2.8 and f22 demonstrates the significance.

Aperture sizes

A lens is defined by two factors, its focal length and maximum aperture, e.g. 100 mm (focal length) f2 (maximum aperture).

'The 'f' number of an optical system is the ratio of the system's focal length to the diameter of the entrance pupil' (Wikipedia) (**Figure 12**). Simply this is the maximum diameter of the usable part of the lens. For example, a 100 mm f2 lens will have a workable lens diameter of 100/2 = 50 mm. A 100 mm f4 lens will have a workable diameter of 100/4 = 25 mm. The latter lens will obviously be smaller and therefore cheaper to manufacture.

Wide aperture lenses such as f2 were more necessary in film days, but current sensors with their low light sensitivity renders this less

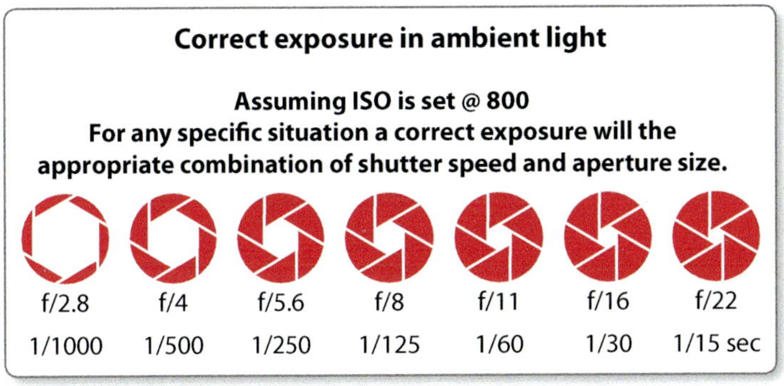

Figure 9 Aperture and shutter speeds.

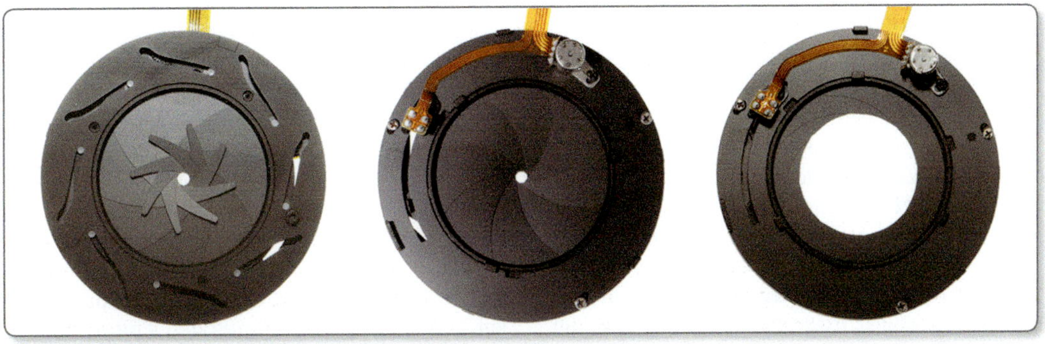

Figure 10 Modern electronically controlled aperture structure.

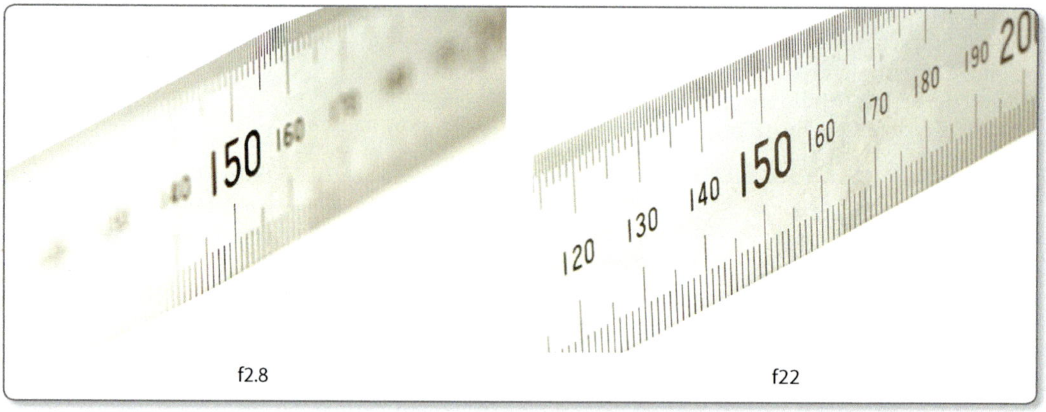

Figure 11 Depth of field (DoF) at large f2.8 and small f22 apertures using 100 mm macro lens.

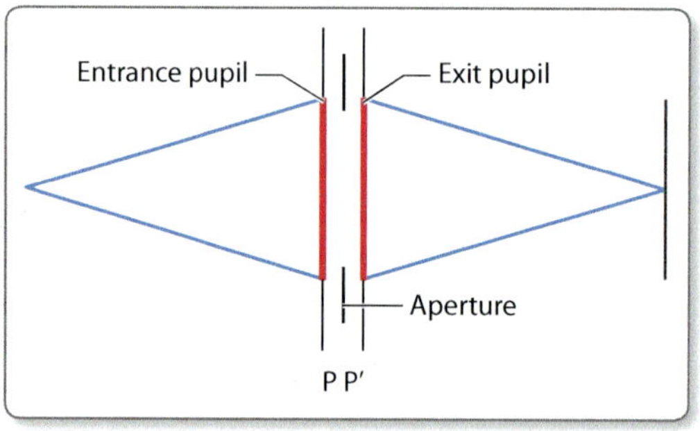

Figure 12 Maximum aperture calculation.

necessary today as ISO changes can be made at any time.

Early lenses incorporated mechanical diaphragms with click stops separating apertures and a fixed ratio (1:2) between the resultant areas. Current lenses have electronically controlled diaphragms which are infinitely variable, and although 'f' values are shown in the display, the relationship from one to another is not known.

The appropriate lens and flash systems for dental photography will be covered in depth in subsequent chapters but the flash function itself will be covered below.

With reference to the aperture and its relation to depth of field (DoF), for close-up clinical work an aperture of f22 will be advocated. This is a very small diameter opening and in combination with a low ISO setting, a very long shutter speed would be required rendering a hand-held camera system impractical. In view of this, an appropriate flash system is recommended.

From **Figure 13**, it is obvious that the typical flash unit integral to most cameras will not illuminate a subject close to the lens and a flash system fitting on or around the lens is recommended.

Flash system function

External flash systems incorporate a power pack which fires the flash tube when the camera shutter is operated. Prior to the 1980s most units were discharged fully on each cycle and the correct exposure was calculated either via a simple formula, or the operator purchased a flash meter to measure the output. Every flash unit has a guide number related to an ISO value and referenced to either feet or metres. A typical guide number being 22 in metres for an ISO of 200. For a subject 2 metres away, one divided 2 into 22 = 11 and the operator would select an aperture of f11 on the lens. Some systems had variable outputs, e.g. ½, ¼, ⅛, etc. but the calculations still had to be made.

Automatic flash exposure

Virtually all current flash systems can be automatically controlled, which, in the author's opinion greatly facilitates and simplifies consistent results. Older flash systems for film cameras will not function automatically with digital cameras as their operating system is entirely different.

It is assumed that the ISO has been pre-set. When the shutter is operated a pilot flash (blue) (**see Figure 14**) leaves the flash gun

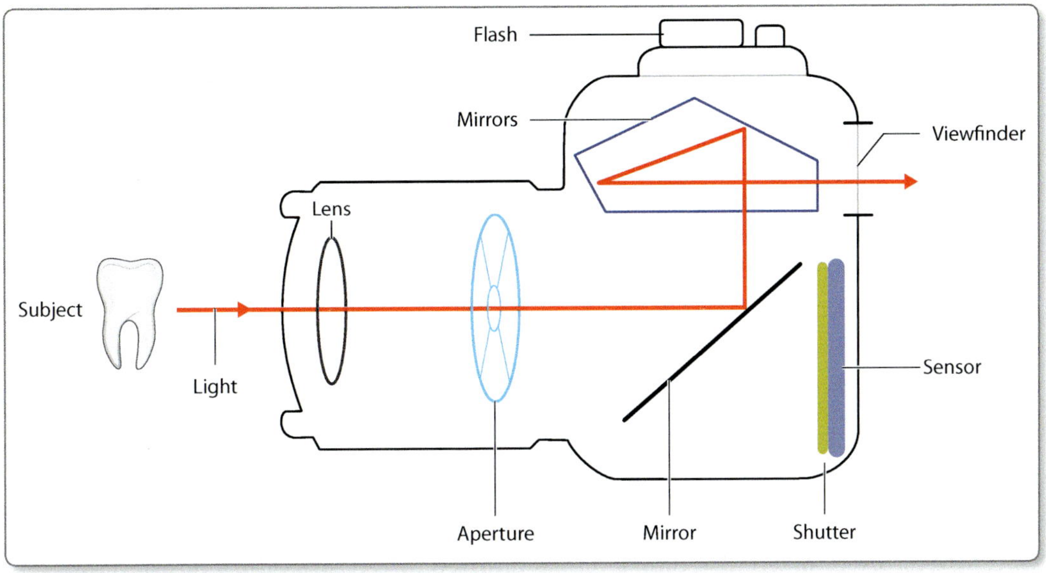

Figure 13 Diagram showing relationship of built-in flash to close-up subject.

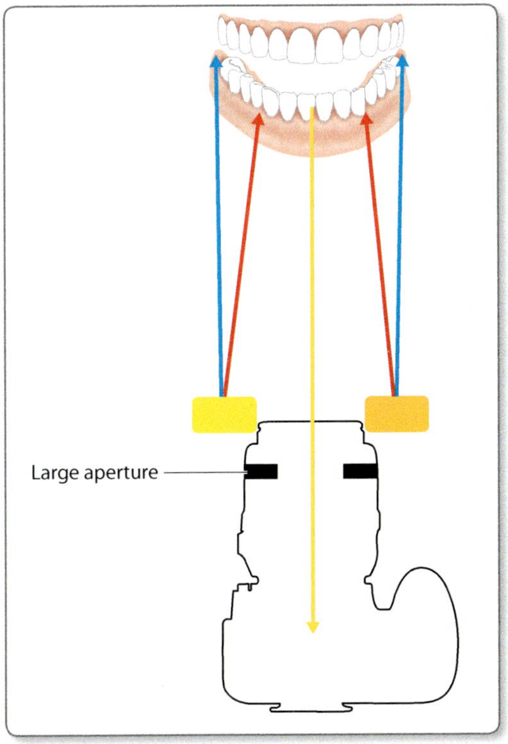

Figure 14a The working of auto through the lens (TTL) flash with current digital cameras.

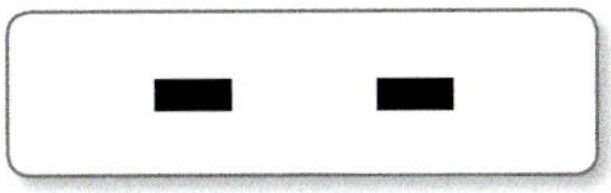

Figure 14b Showing large aperture.

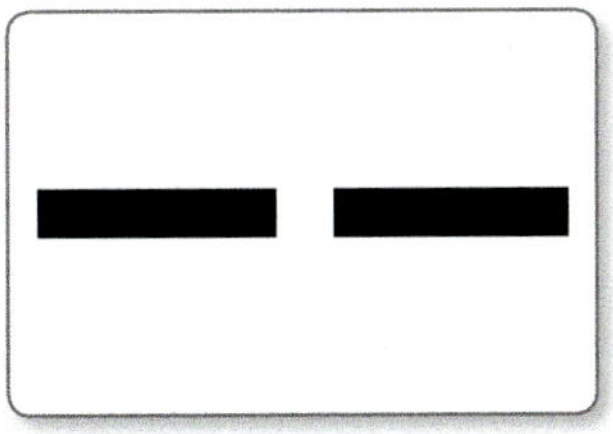

Figure 15 Diagram representing small aperture as opposed to large aperture in Figure 14a.

and a return signal (yellow) enters the camera through the pre-chosen aperture. The return signal is measured by the camera's computer which then calculates the intensity/duration of the exposing flash (red) to ensure a correctly exposed image. This cycle takes approximately 20/1,000,000 seconds.

Figure 14 shows a large aperture; if the operator chooses a smaller aperture, the flash duration would increase appropriately (**Figure 15**).

The major advantage of this system is the power unit is not fully discharged for every exposure and therefore allows rapid subsequent photographs, however, if an attempt is made to take a picture when there is insufficient power, the result can be underexposure, or a system lock up. In the latter instance the answer is to switch the camera off and on again and for the former, allow the flash to re-charge and check the 'ready' light is illuminated.

Film sensitivity (ISO)

ISO numbers refer to the sensitivity of the sensor and have been directly transposed from film.

Films vary in their sensitivity to light, as expressed by their ISO film speed. The higher "the ISO number, the 'faster' the film and the less light you need to take a picture. Fast films of ISO 400, 800 and higher are recommended for dim lighting or fast action such as sports photography."

With film cameras one needed to buy the correct film for a given situation, now with digital sensors, the sensitivity can be changed within the camera.

The term ISO is often erroneously equated to 'International Standards Organisation.' This 'body' per se, does not exist! ISO standards were set by the 'International Organization for Standardization' which would have different acronyms in different languages (IOS in English and OIN in French for Organisation Internationale de Normalisation.) In view of this, the organisation decided to give it the short form ISO. ISO is derived from the Greek isos, meaning equal.

This body, however, did set the standards for film/sensor settings.

The lower the ISO, the higher the quality of the image, and for dental photography a setting of 200 can be considered the norm, ISO sensitivity normally starting at 100.

Focal plane shutter

The shutter keeping light away from the sensor is not a simple open/closed structure but consists of metal, previously cloth, curtains moving in sequence across the focal plane. In practice, particularly at higher shutter speeds, the total surface area of the sensor is not completely exposed at any given time. However brief the shutter setting, e.g. 1/1,000 of a second, it is slow in comparison to electronic flash of 1/20,000 sec. or faster. Therefore, it is essential when using flash, a shutter speed is selected when the whole surface area of the sensor is exposed to the brief duration of the flash (**Figure 16**). This is known as the flash synchronisation speed and fully discussed in Chapter 4.

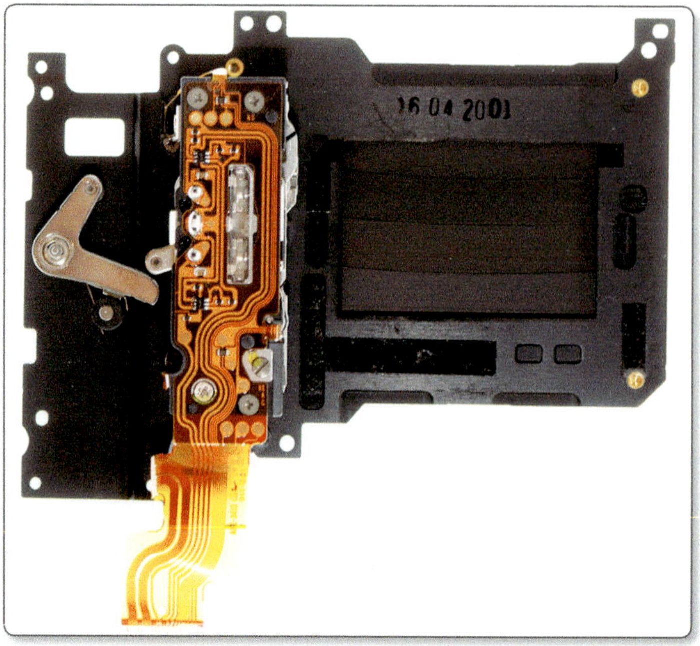

Figure 16 Electronic focal plane shutter assembly.

Flash synchronisation speed

All manufacturers have a recommended shutter speed when electronic flash is used, and they differ from make to make. The function and importance will be discussed where appropriate.

White balance

The white balance (WB) setting control allows the user to pre-set the sensor to render colours accurately according to the source of illumination. Whilst the human eye/brain will generally determine the correct colour of an object however it is illuminated, the camera sensor is not that accurate, and the WB should be pre-set to the light source as appropriate (**Figure 17**).

In the clinical situation virtually all the photography will involve the use of electronic flash and the appropriate WB should be pre-set to Flash ⚡.

One can of course choose 'AUTO' (AWB) when the camera will generally determine an appropriate setting.

Camera modes

All modern DSLR cameras offer Mode settings. These are features which the operator can choose according to the shooting situation. They will be introduced here and expanded upon where necessary.

There is some variation in terminology between manufacturers and variations in options between models from the same manufacturer. Generally according to the mode selected, the operator will pre-set some information, such as ISO and WB and the camera will select the remainder of the operating cycle.

Nikon

Mode selected	Shutter speed	Aperture
P (programmed auto)	Selected by camera	Selected by camera
S (shutter-priority auto)	Selected by photographer	Selected by camera
A (aperture-priority auto)	Selected by camera	Selected by photographer
M (manual)	Selected by photographer	Selected by photographer

Mode selected	Shutter speed	Aperture
P (programmed auto)	Selected by camera	Selected by camera

In this mode, the operator will initially select the ISO and WB and the camera will select the appropriate combination of shutter speed and aperture. Usually aiming for a shutter speed that will lessen the chance of camera shake. The operator will also have a choice of selecting manual or auto focus.

Mode selected	Shutter speed	Aperture
S (shutter-priority auto)	Selected by photographer	Selected by camera

In situations where the shutter speed is of optimum importance, e.g. nature and sports photography, the operator will pre-select the

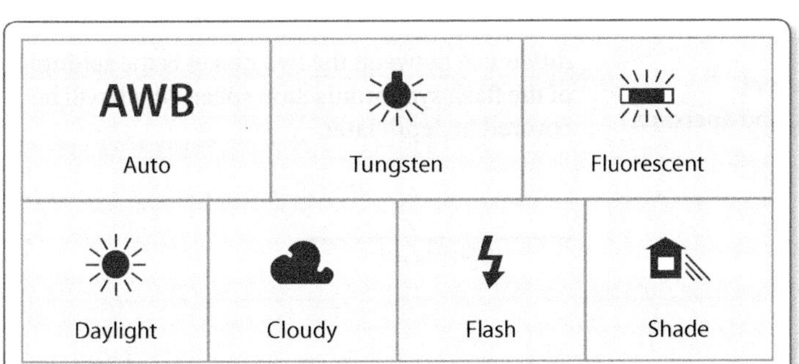

Figure 17 White balance (WB) options.

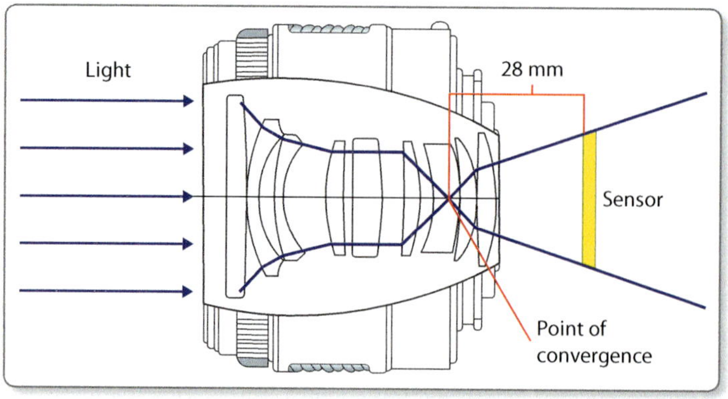

Figure 2 Modern lens construction with 28 mm focal length.

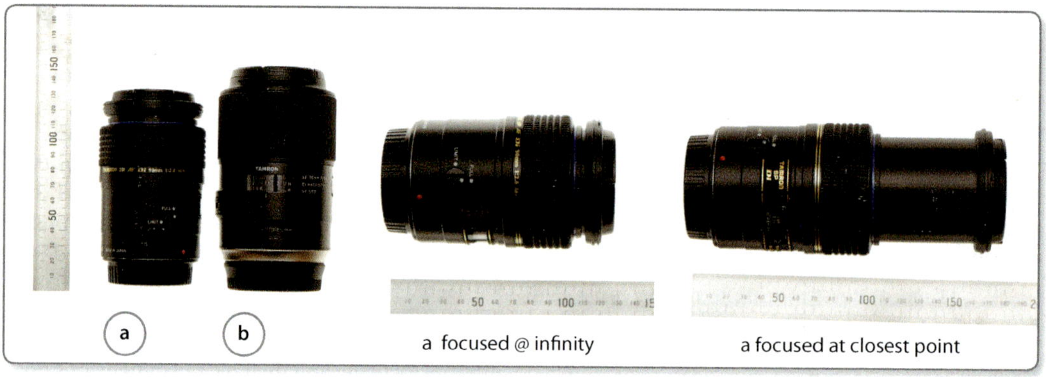

Figure 3 Tamron 90 mm macro lenses. (a) Nonstabilised lens, (b) Stabilised lens.

mount to the subject is 100 mm. The stabilised version with internal focusing will be 150 mm from the subject to give an equivalent sized image.

Working distance is critically important in intraoral photography. Invariably the light source is on or around the lens, therefore the camera system must be far enough away to allow illumination of the buccal corridor, and where close up or facial photography is concerned the distance should allow a natural perspective. In practical terms the minimum focal length of 85 mm on a full frame camera and in theory 60 mm and above on a crop sensor camera. However, the shorter working distance using a 60 mm lens does cause a perspective problem (see **Figures 4** and **5**). If oral surgery photography is considered, the extra working distance afforded by 100 mm or 105 mm lenses is essential and the use of any bracket system placing the flash heads forward of the lens would be totally impractical (**Figure 6**).

Angle of view

The focal length also determines the angle of view: The longer the focal length, the narrower the field of view. Nearly all the current macro lenses were designed for 35 mm film cameras and the angle of view effectively changes if these lenses are used on smaller format cameras. For example, a 100 mm lens on a full frame sensor has a 20° field of view but only 13° on the smaller cropped APS-C sensor (Advance Photo System Type) (**Figures 4** and **5**).

Whilst there is perhaps a minimal difference using these lenses on facial views (**Figure 4**), the shorter working distance using the 60 mm lens proves more significant in the close-up situation (see **Figure 5**).

Whilst images from either 60 mm or 100 mm lenses would be considered suitable for record purposes, it would be essential for ONE focal length lens to be used for consistency in perspective.

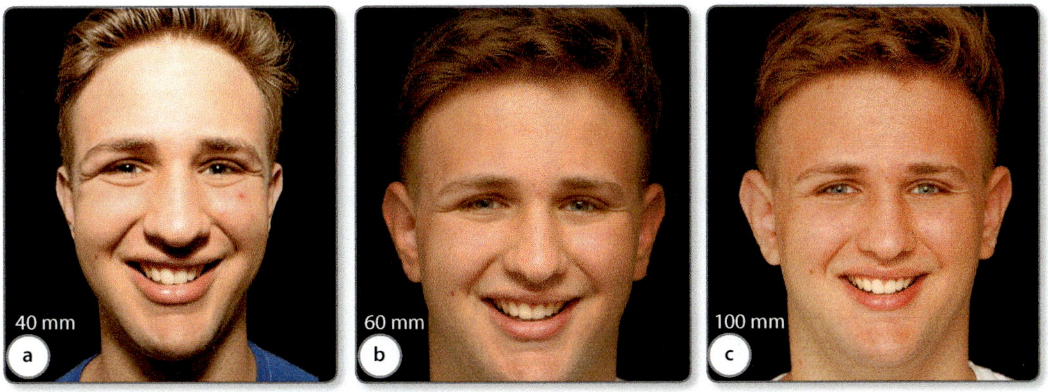

Figure 4 Facial views with (a) 40 mm, (b) 60 mm, and (c) 100 mm lenses on a crop sensor camera demonstrating the perspective change with different working distances when achieving similar sized images.

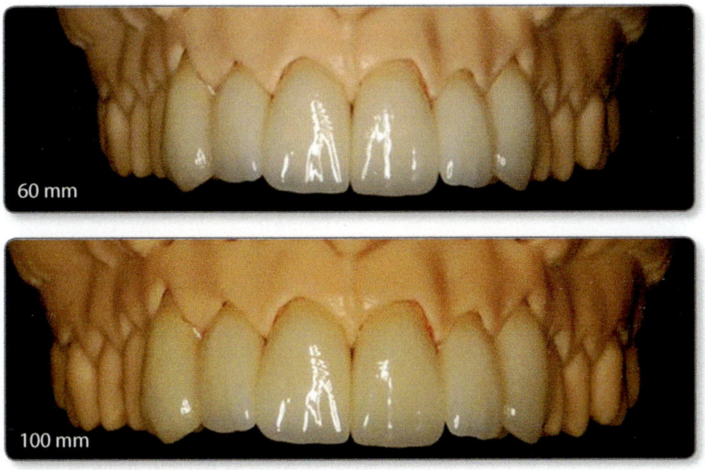

Figure 5 Close-up photographs with 60 mm and 100 mm lens.

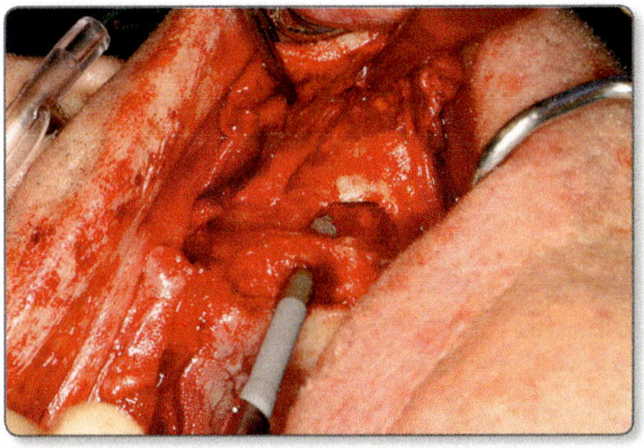

Figure 6 Zygomatic implant placement. Canon 100 mm lens + MR 14 EX II Flash.
(*Courtesy:* Dr Andrew Dawood surgeon photograph by the author)

Magnification ratio

Magnification ratio is the relationship between the size of the subject and the actual size of the image on the film or sensor (**Figure 7**).

Most if not all current macro lenses used on cropped sensor digital single-lens reflex (DSLR) cameras were originally designed for use with 35 mm film and currently full frame digital sensor cameras, and the close-up ratios, in yellow (in **Figure 7**), refer to that format. These ratios refer to the size of the original subject to the size of its image on the sensor. At 1:2 on a full frame sensor, the image would be exactly half-life size. To achieve an equivalent field of view on

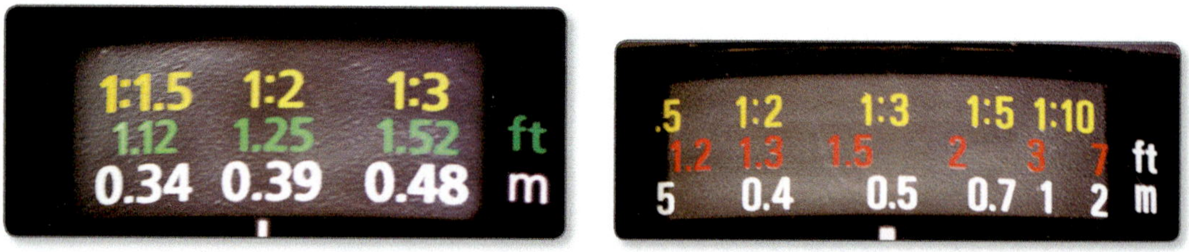

Figure 7 Typical views of lens barrels showing magnification ratios in yellow.

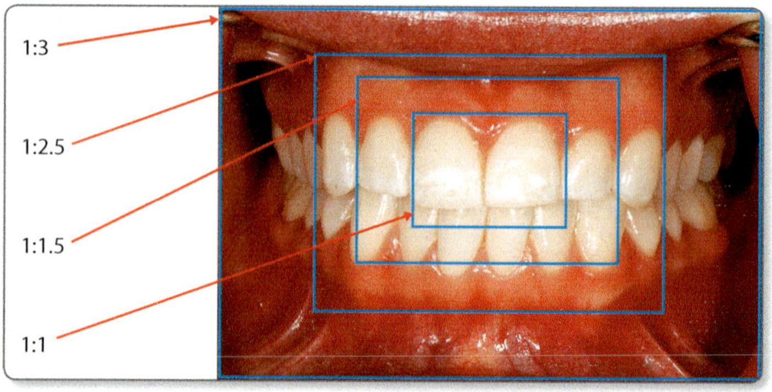

Figure 8 Areas covered by ratios set in yellow on lens fitted to a cropped sensor camera.

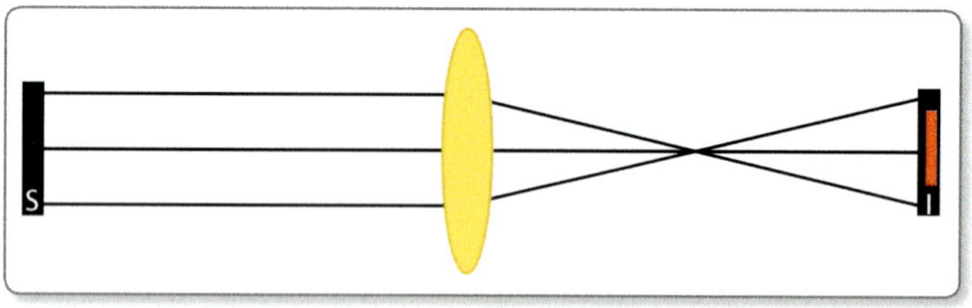

Figure 9 Diagram showing areas covered by full frame and cropped sensor cameras.

a cropped sensor camera the ratio would need to be set at 1:3.

Pre selecting a ratio and moving the camera until focus is achieved fixes the camera to subject distance and ensures consistency of image size. On a cropped sensor camera presetting the following values will achieve the approximate fields of view (**Figure 8**).

Consider 100 mm macro lens fitted to a full frame DSLR camera focussed to produce a 1:1 image, as in **Figure 9** where subject 'S' is the same size as image 'I.' If the same lens is fitted to a DSLR with an APS-C (smaller sensor) only approximately two-thirds of the original subject will be captured on the smaller sensor (RED in **Figure 9**).

Figure 10 shows the approximate difference between a view of the anterior teeth at 1:1 on a full frame camera and the same lens set at 1:1 on an APS-C sensor. This difference is known as the 'CROP FACTOR' and is 1.5× with Nikon and 1.6× with Canon. This can also be interpreted as follows. A 100 mm focal length lens designed for a full frame camera, if placed on a camera with an APS-C sensor it will have the same effect as placing a 150/160 mm lens on the full frame system. This can be an advantage with close-up photography as the working distance is increased, but occasionally the increased working distance for taking full faces can result with 'space' difficulties in very small surgeries.

Aperture

The function of the aperture in relation to exposure was covered in Chapter 1; however, the aperture size is of great importance especially in close-up photography as it also controls the depth of field (DoF).

In a large percentage of dental photographic images, the subject size approaches the actual size of the image on the sensor (magnification ratio). At these extremes the DoF is measured in millimetres.

Depth of field

Depth of field is the distance between objects closest to and the furthest from the lens, giving an image which the eye will accept as being 'in focus,' and refers to objects in front of the lens.

Consider **Figure 11** which represents 'RED,' 'BLACK' and 'BLUE' pin size subjects to the left of the lens. As a lens has only one specific point of focus only the RED subject will be in focus at the focal plane and the BLACK and BLUE points will be represented as circles. If these circles are

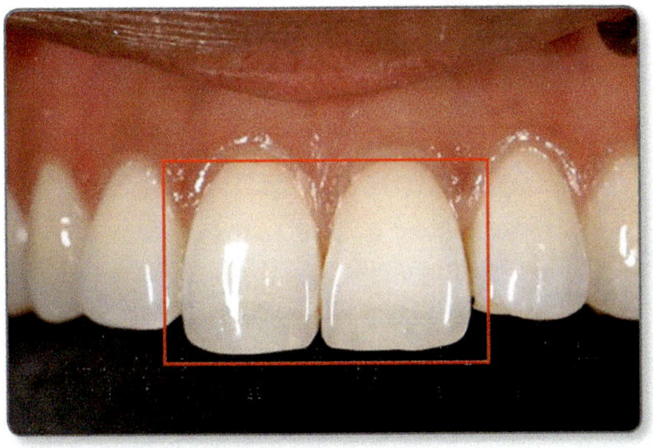

Figure 10 Difference between a view of the anterior teeth at 1:1 on a full frame camera and the same lens set at 1:1 on an advanced photo system type-C sensor (APS-C).

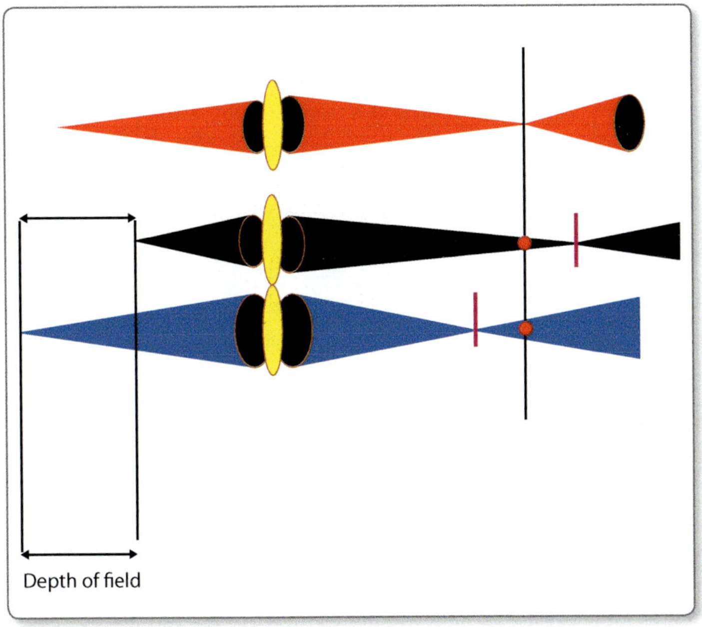

Figure 11 Depth of field.

below a certain size, the eye will accept them as being 'in focus.' For cropped sensor cameras it is 1/20 mm and 1/30 mm for full frame cameras. This is referred to as, 'the circle of confusion.' Assuming these parameters are met in the diagram, the distance between the two vertical black lines represents the DoF, and for the technically minded the distance between the two red lines is referred to as the depth of focus and is behind the lens.

How aperture changes affects depth of field

When the aperture is reduced in size the light path angle is reduced and the range of 'circle of confusion' acceptability is increased (see **Figure 12**).

In **Figure 12**, top diagram, only 'B' would be in acceptable focus as 'A' and 'C' would be represented as out of focus circles, in the lower diagram these circles are reduced in size and acceptable to the eye. The distance A to C being the 'depth of field.'

Optical stabilisation

One of the most common causes of image degradation is that of 'CAMERA SHAKE,' i.e. inadvertent movement of the camera assembly at the point of operating the shutter. In general photography using ambient light, the operator would try to use an aperture allowing a suitable shutter speed to minimise this eventuality. Rule of thumb being, 'use a shutter speed numerically equivalent to the focal length of the lens." 100 mm use 1/100 seconds; 200 mm use 1/200 seconds, etc. or faster.

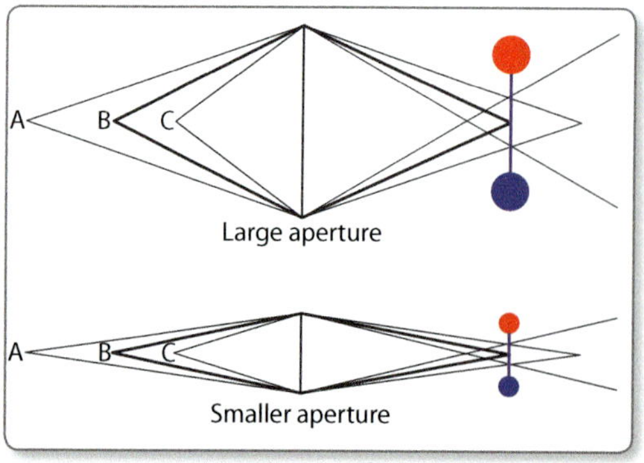

Figure 12 Diagram showing how reduction of aperture size increases depth of field.

Many current lenses now incorporate some form of image stabilisation by using floating optics to compensate for slight camera body movement. Manufacturers have different terms for this function:

- Nikon uses VR (vibration reduction)
- Canon uses IS (image stabilisation)
- Sigma uses OS (optical stabilisation)
- Tamron uses VC (vibration control)

Olympus having ceased production of full frame or cropped sensor single-lens reflex cameras, has gone in another direction and built vibration control into the camera with the sensor being 'movable.' Thus, the camera has the stability function and the facility is not required for any lens used.

Do you need optical stabilisation for dental photography?

In short, the answer is, 'No!' In the clinical situation utilising electronic flash, the duration of the flash is so brief compared with the shutter speed, any form of stabilisation is unnecessary. However, using a macro lens for close-up work in daylight, e.g. flower or insect photography, stabilisation would be beneficial. Of course, the clinical set up is ideal for this situation.

Is there a choice?

Currently the Sigma 105 mm macro is only available in a stabilised version, as is the Nikon 105 mm.

Canon currently produce 100 mm stabilised and nonstabilised versions.

Tamron also run 90 mm macro lenses in both formats.

As far the operator is concerned, the function is a switchable option, the penalty is a significantly heavier lens and invariably more expensive.

Autofocus

As photographic systems have progressed over the last 150–200 years, manufacturers have strived to simplify camera use and simultaneously achieve higher quality results. Simply the autofocus function enables the camera lens to focus automatically on the subject so that the final image is sharp. The pitfalls and use or nonuse of autofocus in relation to dental photography will be discussed in Chapter 4.

3 Lighting systems

Introduction

This chapter will cover lighting for intra-/peri-oral situations using both basic and more complex systems. Facial photography will be discussed in Chapter 8. In view of the proximity of camera to subject with intra- and peri-oral photography it is essential that any illumination system is placed either on (axial) or near the lens. Invariably the most satisfactory method is electronic flash which will be discussed here together with some alternative systems.

Axial illumination

There is currently a multitude of systems available with a variety of light sources and extreme price ranges. Those discussed in the text will have been used by the author and/or have full UK support. In the author's experience some comparatively very cheap flash systems have proved unreliable, particularly in the long-term or in heavy usage situations such as orthodontic practices.

Originally, 'on the lens' illumination was provided by a true 'ring flash' with a circular flash tube (see Figure 32 of Chapter 6). Current 'ring flash' systems generally utilise two small flash tubes, the advantage being the ability to vary the output or eliminate one tube to create uneven lighting or reduce shadowing in selected circumstances. One true ring flash is currently produced by Lester Dine in the US (see **Figure 1**); however, it is normally sold as a combination 'ring and point system' (see **Figure 2**).

Compatibility

Manufacturers obviously want you to purchase their own accessories which are generally more expensive than third party 'equivalents,' which except for the Metz 15MS-1, are specific for one make. Canon accessories are only fully compatible with Canon equipment and similarly Nikon with Nikon. Current third-party accessories may not function completely with the latest camera bodies. Note the differences in the hot shoe contacts of the Nikon **Figure 3** and Canon **Figure 4**. In addition, note the difference between the Canon 200D hot shoe **Figure 4** and its current successor the 250D **Figure 5** (August 2019).

The revised configuration renders existing third party flash accessories for Canon partially or totally incompatible with the latest body.

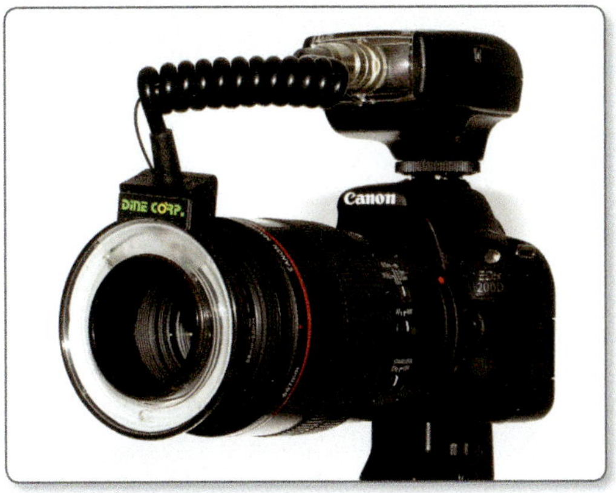

Figure 1 Lester Dine true ring flash.

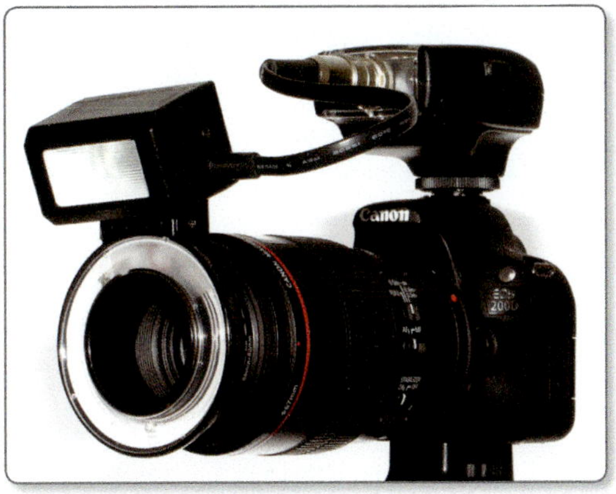

Figure 2 Lester Dine combination flash.

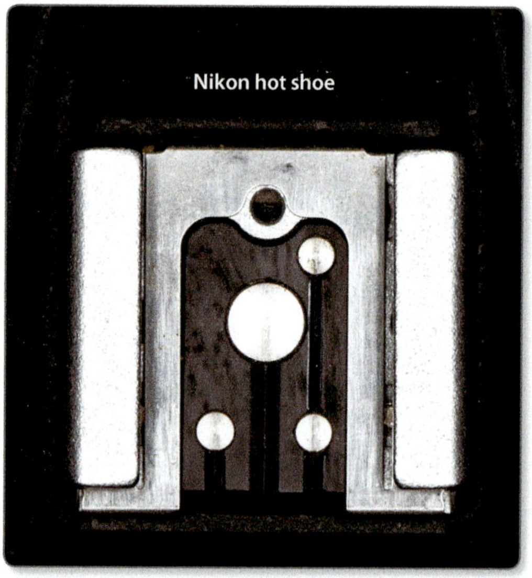

Figure 3 Nikon hot shoe.

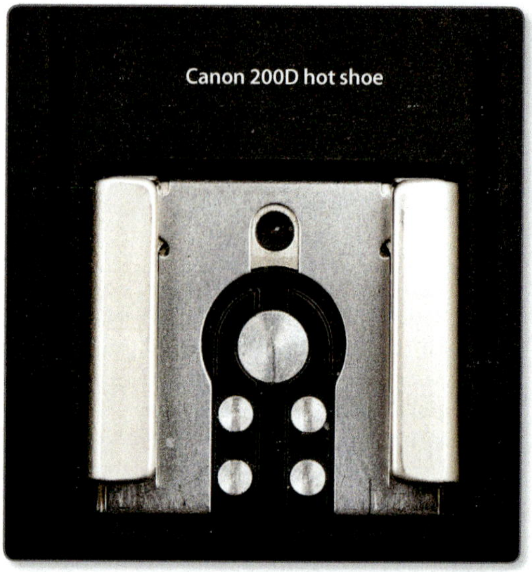

Figure 4 Typical Canon hot shoe.

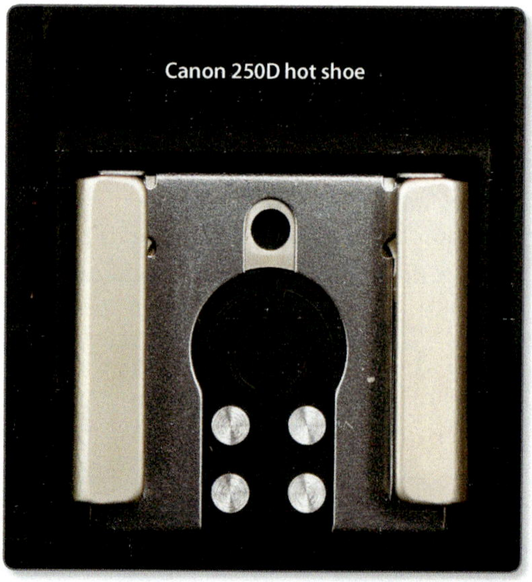

Figure 5 Latest Canon hot shoe.

Ring flash

The mainstream 'ring flash' units by Canon, Nissin, Kenro, and Metz all utilise two small flash units in one mount (see **Figures 6a** to **c**). Their major advantage is they are always pointing in the right direction and invariably illuminate the buccal corridor on full arch anterior views. Major disadvantages, some consider the illumination to be on the flat side, the other being harsh reflections on close-up anterior views (see Figures 2 and 3 of Chapter 7).

The lightest 'ring flash' unit with full Through The Lens metering (TTL) function is the Metz 15MS-1 (**Figure 7**) which does not have a separate wired power pack. It utilises two AAA batteries unlike the other flash systems which use four AA cells. Whilst all other 'third party' flash systems are specific to one make; these units can be individually programmed for different manufacturers. As they do not have a power pack with a physical hot shoe connection they rely on a wireless/optical trigger from the 'host' camera's flash; and in order to function fully with TTL metering a compatible body is required. The MS-1 responds to a coded infra-red-light signal emitted from the camera's own flash and utilises a clip-on filter which prevents the camera's flash influencing the exposure. Unfortunately, this automatic metering function is not available with many low-end entry level digital single-lens reflexes (DSLRs) and compatibility must be checked prior to purchase. However, for existing systems the MS-1 can be triggered by purchasing a small compatible flash gun such as the Canon EL 100 (**Figure 8**) to function with Canon cameras or appropriate Metz M400 designated for Nikon or Canon and thus maintain full TTL automatic metering.

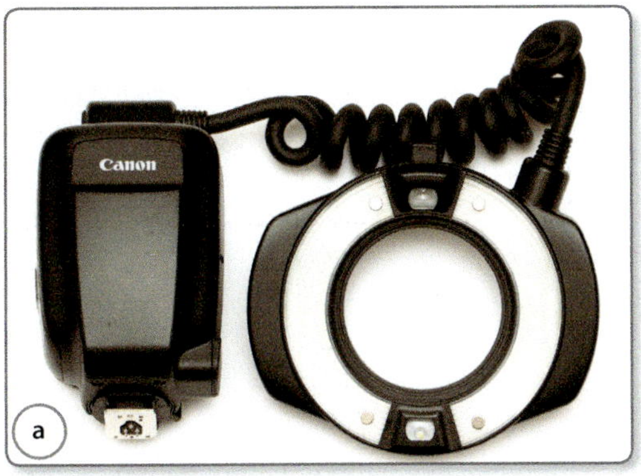

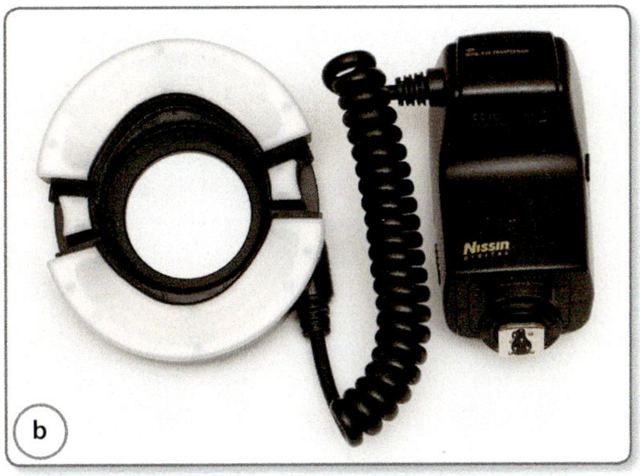

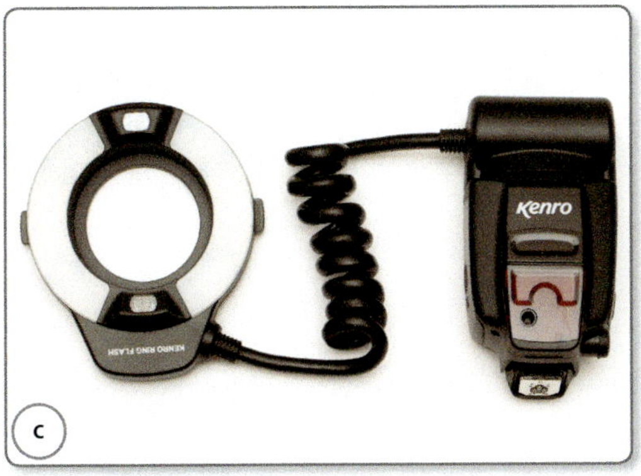

Figure 6 Typical ring flash units with power packs. (a) Canon MR EX II, (b) Nissin MF–18, (c) Kenro KLF 201.

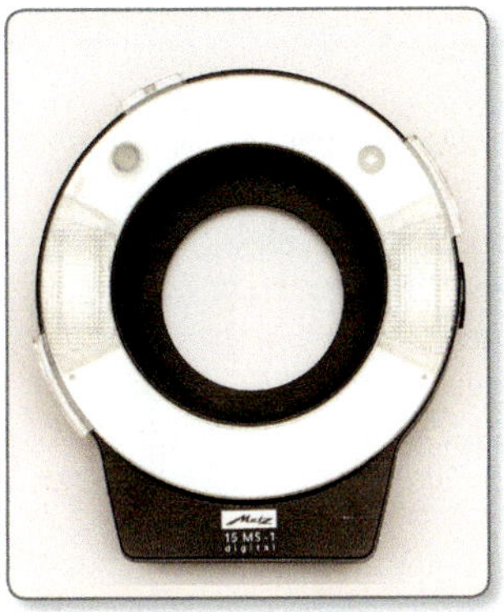

Figure 7 Metz 15MS-1 flash.

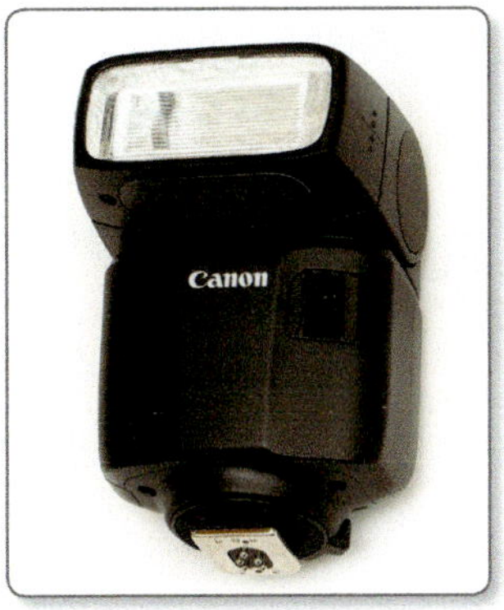

Figure 8 Canon EL 100 flash.

When considering purchasing a new body together with a third party flash such as the Metz MS-1, it is far cheaper to purchase a compatible body, the Canon 800D for example, from the outset rather than buying accessories to enable one piece of equipment 'to talk' to another! See **Figures 9** and **10**. When using an accessory flash to trigger the Metz MS-1 it can be pointed away as shown in **Figure 11** or used with the Metz filter as in **Figure 12**.

The MS-1 flash can however be triggered by any built-in camera flash by setting it in 'SERVO' mode. This means that the flash will fire at the manually set power output and correct exposure will need to be determined by experiment. Another option is to purchase a PC cable to

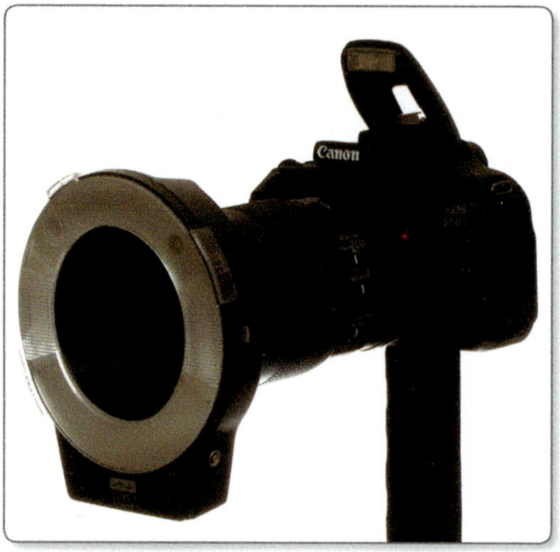

Figure 9 Canon 800D + Metz MS-1 flash.

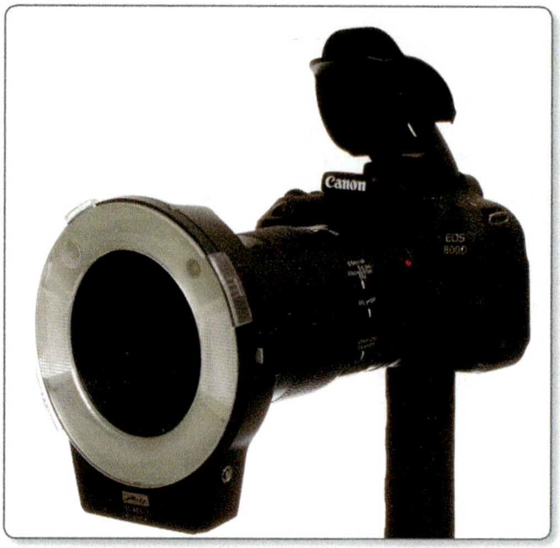

Figure 10 Metz filter on camera flash Canon 800D.

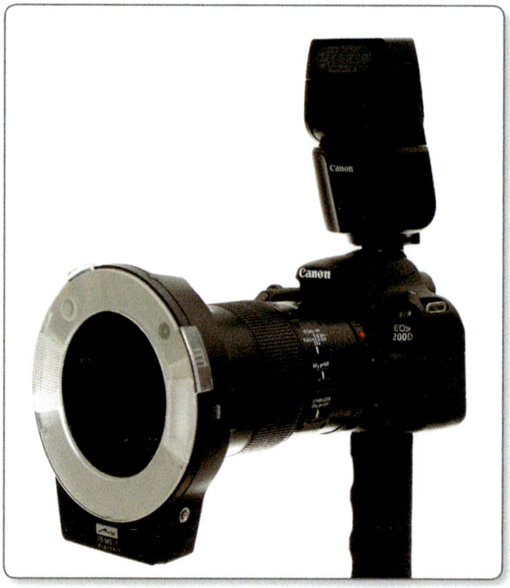

Figure 11 Canon 200D + EL 100 flash to trigger Metz MS-1 flash.

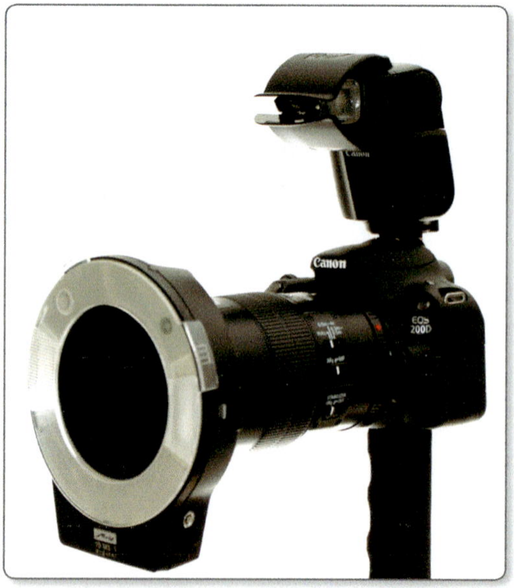

Figure 12 Metz Filter on EL 100 flash to trigger Metz MS-1 flash.

connect the flash directly to the camera, this time by setting the flash in 'SYNC' mode, this will also lose the TTL function so that trial shots will be needed to establish the correct aperture/ISO combination. As a rough guide, using the flash at full power, and setting the camera in Manual 'M' mode, an ISO of 100 and using an aperture of f22 for close-ups and f8 for faces will generally give excellent results. This is probably the only 'ring flash' with internal reflectors giving the ability to change the angle of illumination.

There is a significant difference between triggering an 'off camera' flash wirelessly to illuminate the subject whilst maintaining automatic exposure control as above and

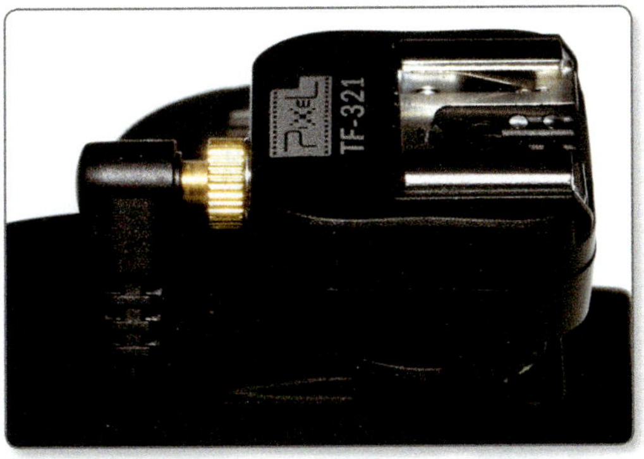

Figure 13 Hot shoe to PC converter for Canon.

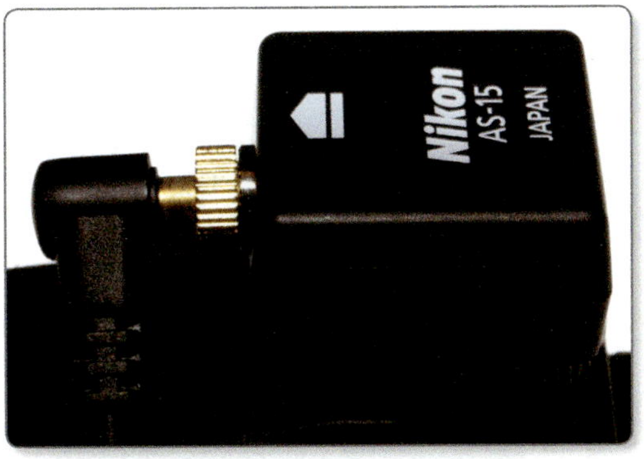

Figure 14 Hot shoe to PC converter for nikon.

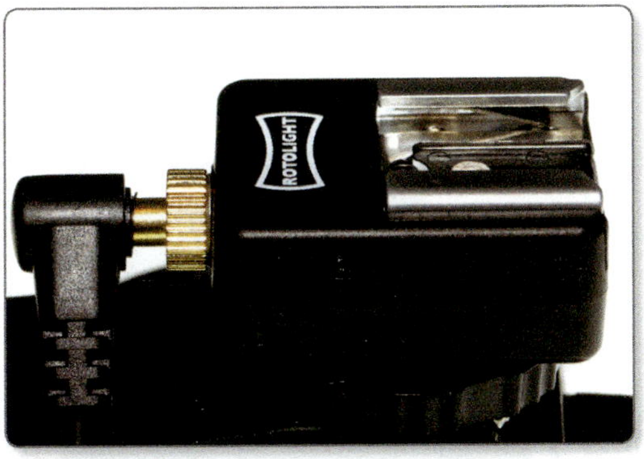

Figure 15 Rotolight universal PC converter.

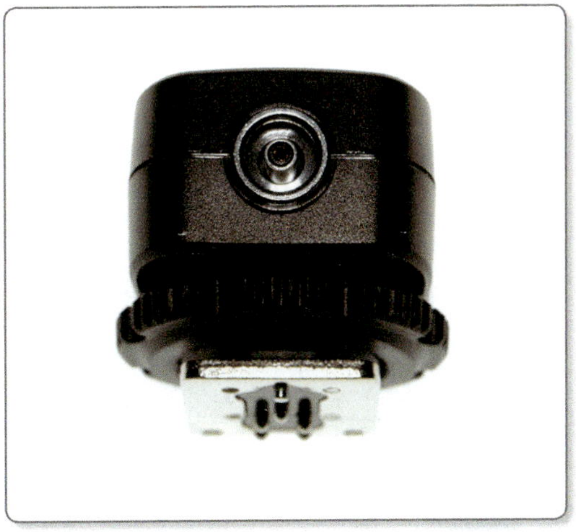

Figure 16 PC socket.

triggering a slave flash to eliminate shadows which will be discussed in a later chapter.

Low end or entry level Canon and Nikon cameras do not have a PC socket to link to external flash units, but a hot-shoe adaptor such as TF-321 (**Figure 13**) for Canon, AS-15 for Nikon (**Figure 14**), and universal by Rotolight© (**Figure 15**) will allow a cable connection to the Metz 15MS-1. In fact, the Nikon AS-15 will work with older Canon cameras but may not work with the latest due to the revised hot shoe configuration (**Figures 16** to **19**).

Combination flash

The Lester Dine RING/POINT unit combines a true RING light with circular flash tube and a single POINT source which can be rotated around the lens. The flash units can only be fired individually and are specific for Nikon and Canon cameras only (**Figure 20**).

Twin flash systems

Many colleagues are now seeking systems to achieve more aesthetic lighting and turning to the versatility of twin flash systems using the flash heads on the lens or on other bracket systems such as: The Owl, Axis, Agnos, Molaris, and PhotoMed. There is also an increasing interest in the use of small soft boxes and bouncers to diffuse the light source. These systems will be introduced here but described in detail in later. The Nikon R1C1 system has a lens mount for two or more SB-R200 small flash units which are triggered wirelessly by either a commander unit mounted in the hot shoe or by the camera's built-in flash depending on the model. The Canon T24/26 system is similar in principle, but the flash heads are tethered to a power pack (see **Figures 21** and **22**).

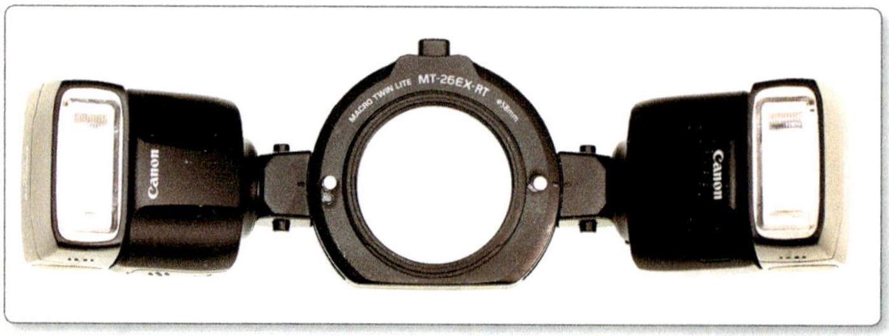

Figure 24 2 EL 100 units on MT 24/26 mount.

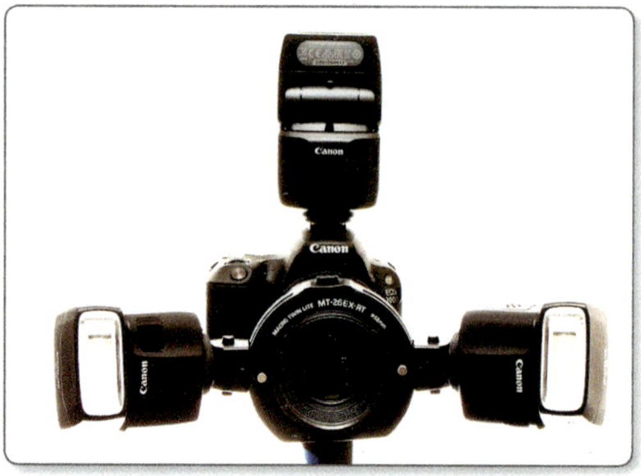

Figure 25 EL 100 unit used as trigger on Canon 200D with 2 EL 100 units on MT 24/26 mount.

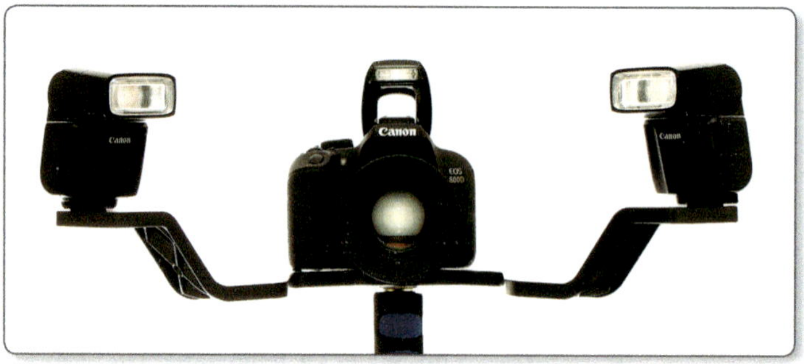

Figure 26 Canon 800D's inbuilt flash triggering EL 100 flashes on Axis bracket.

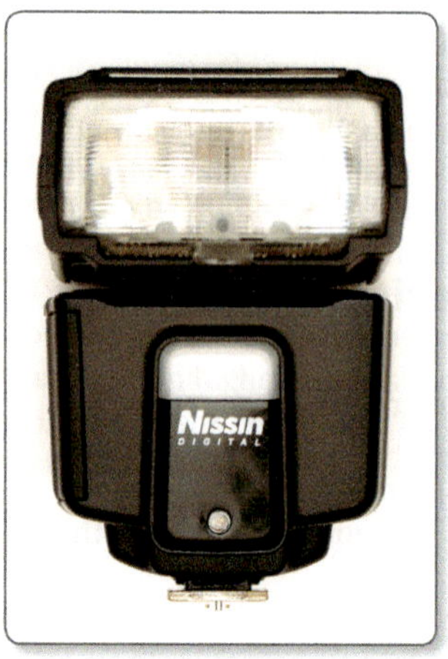

Figure 27 Nissin i40.

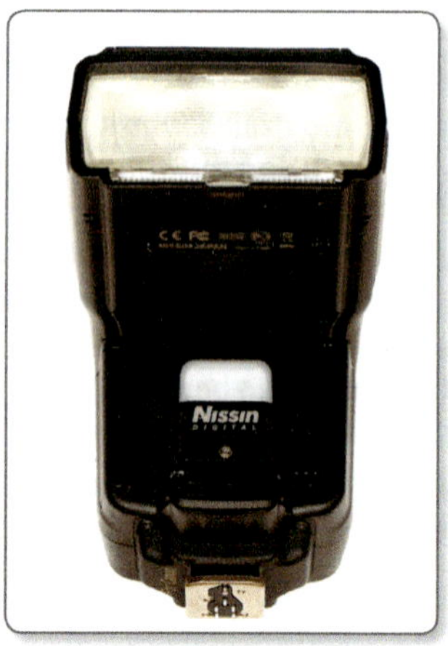

Figure 28 Nissin i60.

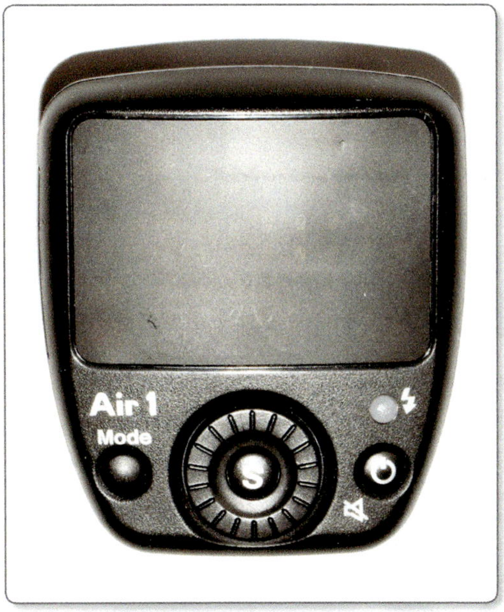

Figure 29 Nissin 'AIR' wireless trigger.

settings. They are manufactured for use with either Nikon SB-R200 flash units or regular flash systems (**Figures 33** and **34**). The Owl offers more flexibility in flash positioning with ball and socket mounts, but this can add to complications!

Agnos

The Axis, PhotoMed, and Molaris brackets have all been designed predominantly for dental photography. Agnos brackets have been manufactured to cover close-up and macro photography in general and currently three models are available. Each design is produced specifically for either the Nikon SB-R200 units or standard flashes. The Scorpion CLASSIC (**Figure 35**) is the heaviest and can be extended as shown in **Figure 35**. In the author's opinion, forward extension of flash units is probably impractical for clinical dentistry, and the smaller and lighter brackets are more convenient (**Figure 36**).

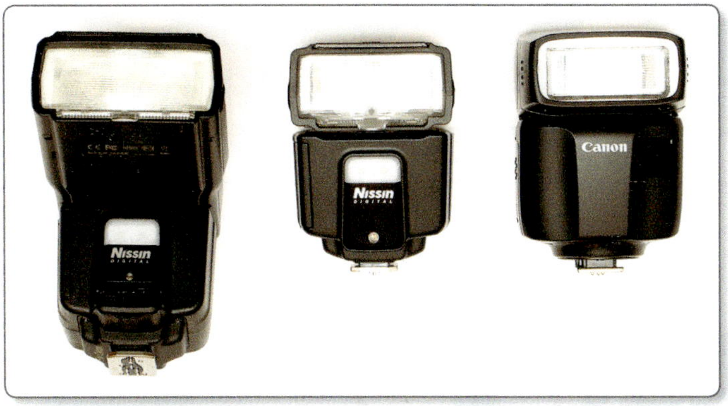

Figure 30 Size comparison Nissin i60, i40, and Canon EL 100 flash units.

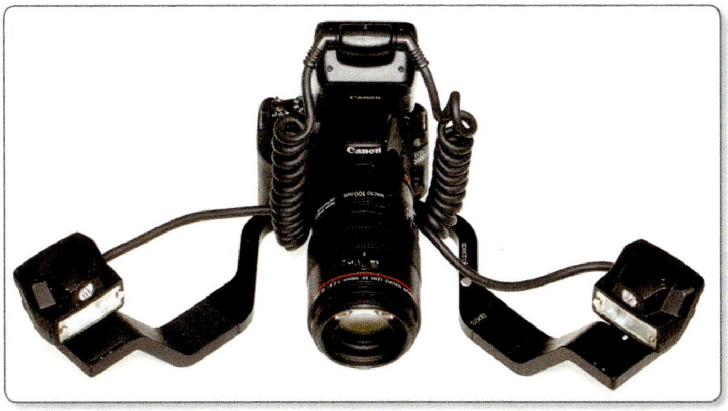

Figure 31 Axis bracket with Canon MT24/26 flash.

All the brackets mentioned are bulky and relatively heavy, the Canon EL 100 flash units use 2 AA cells and are considerably lighter than the Nissin i40 and i60 units which use 4 AA cells.

Lighting systems compared

A model with full upper arch restorations, courtesy Knight Dental Design Laboratory, was set-up as the standard subject to be photographed with a variety of lighting systems. The model position was fixed, and the camera was tripod mounted to give as much consistency and stability as possible. Two camera systems were used, Canon & Nikon. Each was set-up at ISO 200, White Balance (WB) for electronic flash, and an aperture of f22. Flash operation was set to TTL automatic exposure. Canon 100 mm macro and Nikon 105 mm macro lenses were used. The exercise was to compare glare from the flash units, and these can best be described as typical in the current situation and would obviously vary slightly in other cases. The readers will note that whilst automatic exposure was constantly accurate the light output from the flash units varied slightly giving rise to slight colour difference in the final images emphasising the necessity for consistency in equipment to ensure consistency in the results. In addition, there were slight colour casts from some flash accessories.

Figures 40 to 42 and **44 to 49** show typical results using standard 'Ring Flash' systems, incorporating two flash tubes placed routinely at 9 and 3 o'clock. These systems can be considered suitable for most clinical work including surgery (**Figures 50** and **51**). **Figure 43** shows that placing the flash tubes in the 12 and 6 o'clock position and blanking or switching

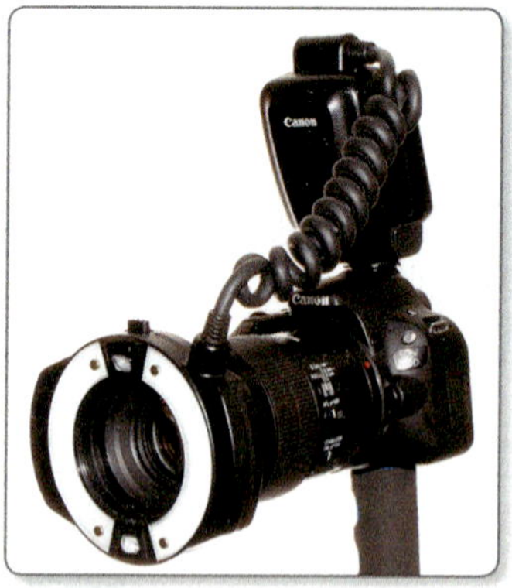

Figure 40 Canon MR EX II flash.

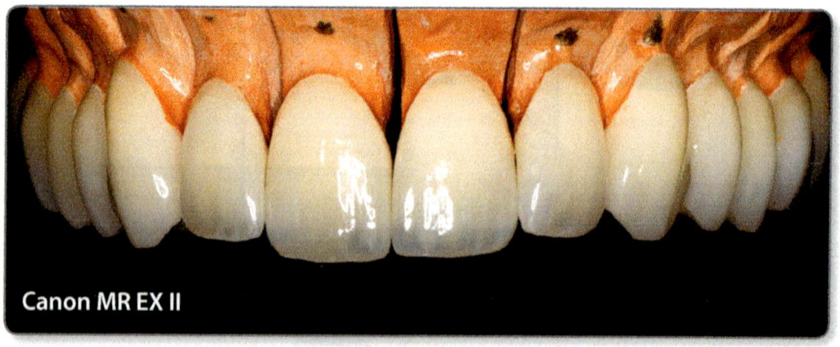

Figure 41 Image taken with MR 14EX II.

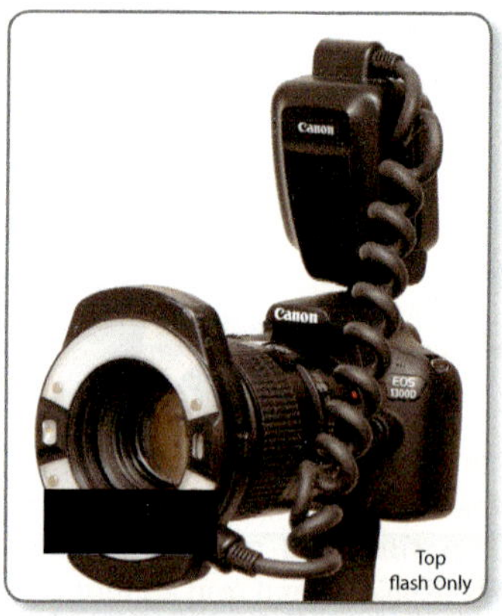

Figure 42 Canon MR EX II with top flash switched on only. Blank for illustrative purpose only.

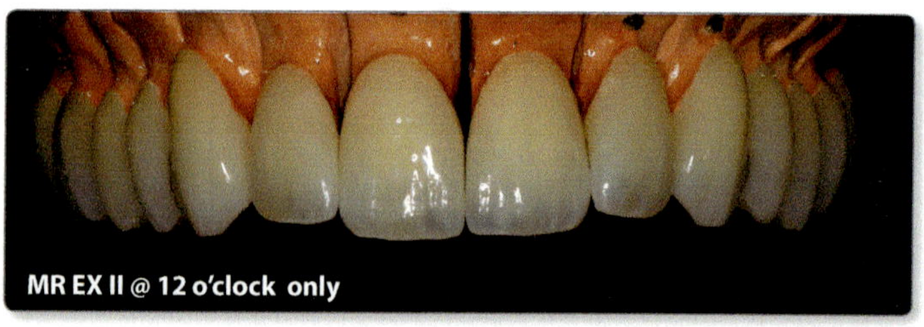

Figure 43 Image taken with flash @ 12 o'clock firing only.

off the lower flash, the incisal translucency is accentuated (**Figure 43**). This image was taken with a Canon flash, it can be assumed that similar results would be achieved with all similar "ring lashes."

Combination flash

For images using Lester Dine ring/point system (see **Figures 52** to **55**).

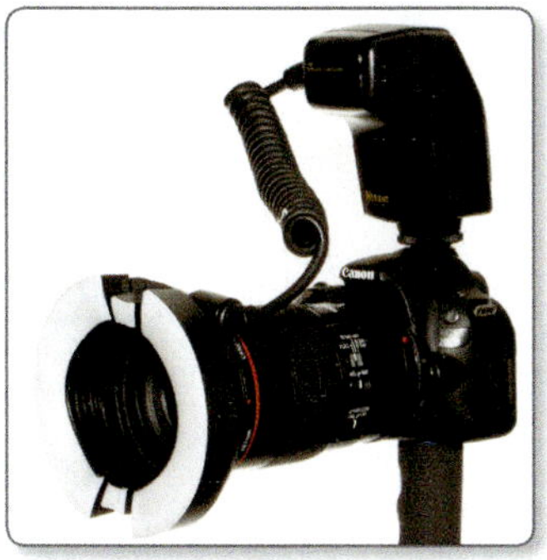

Figure 44 Nissin MF-18.

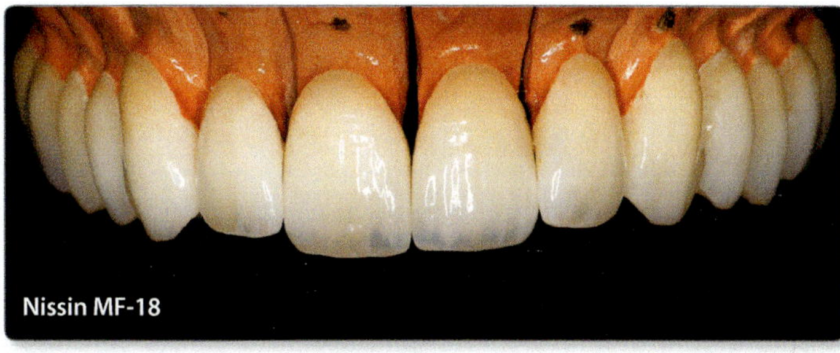

Figure 45 Image taken with Nissin MF-18.

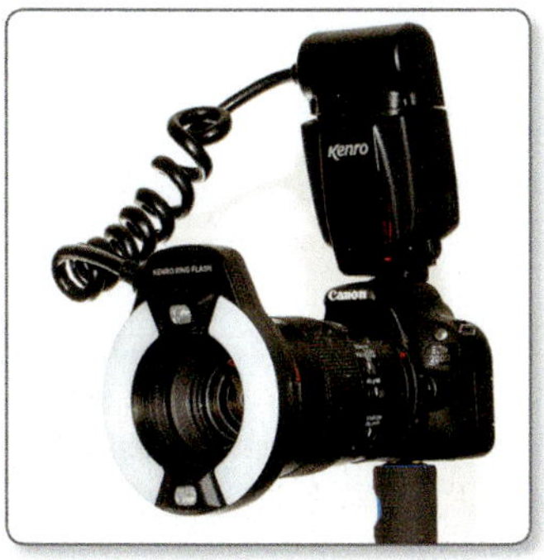

Figure 46 Kenro KFL 201.

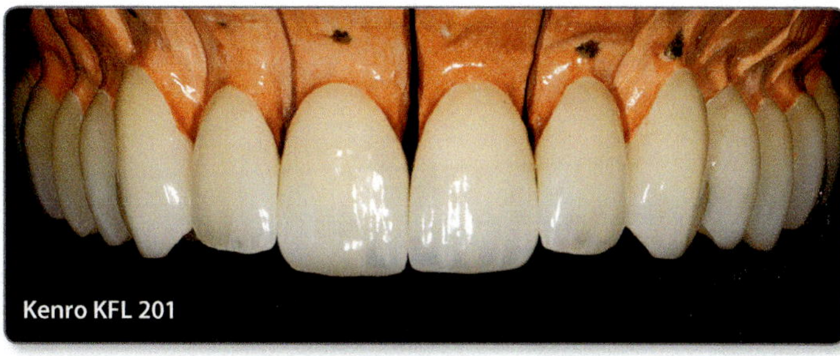

Figure 47 Image taken with Kenro KFL 201.

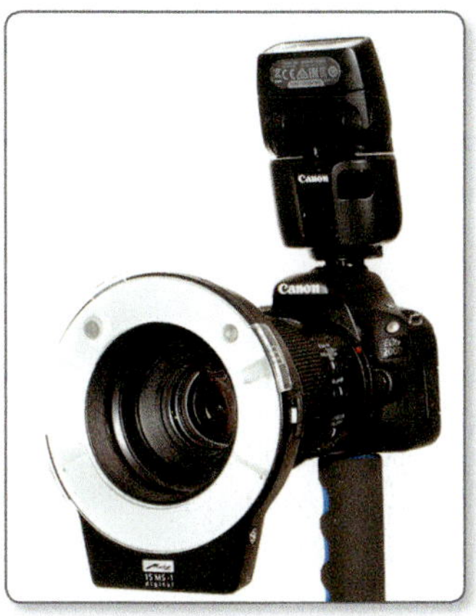

Figure 48 Metz MS-1.

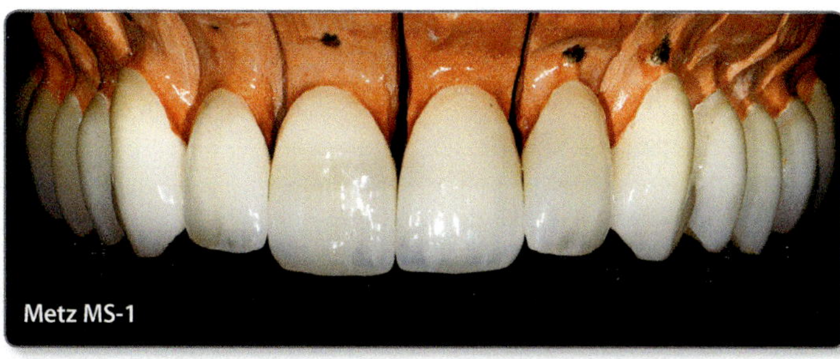

Figure 49 Image taken with Metz MS-1.

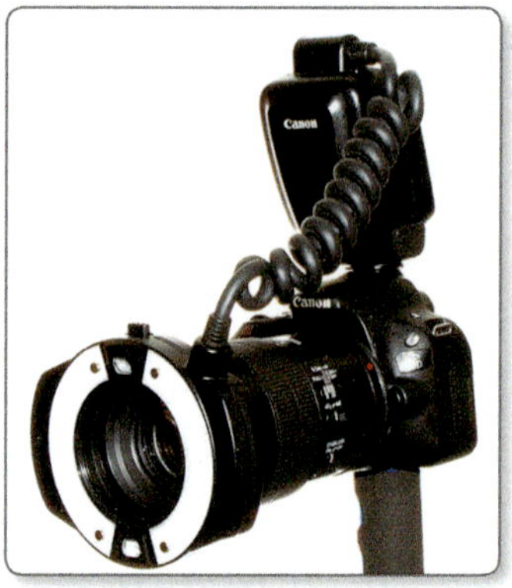

Figure 50 Canon MR EX II system used for Figure 51.

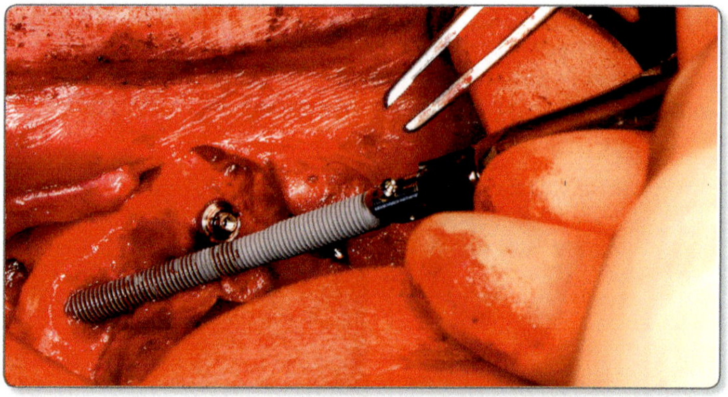

Figure 51 Zygomatic implant placement using set up as Figure 50. (Dr Andrew Dawood); photography (Dr Peter Gordon).

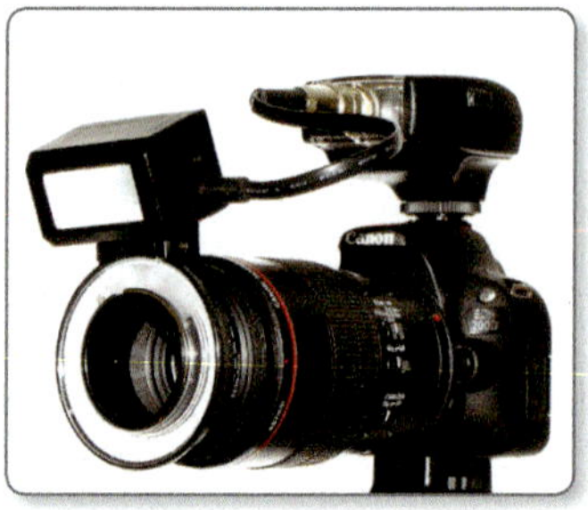

Figure 52 Dine combination flash.

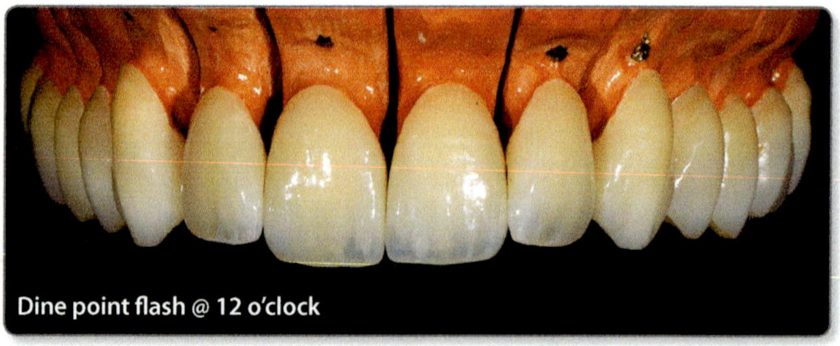

Figure 53 Image taken with point flash @ 12 o'clock.

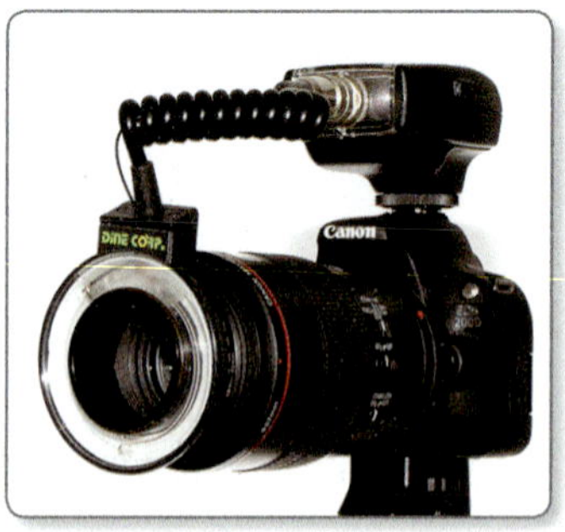

Figure 54 Dine ring flash.

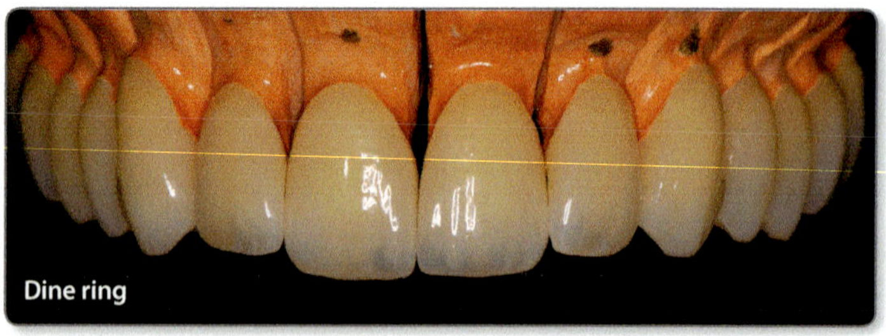

Figure 55 Image taken with Dine ring flash.

Twin flash systems

The instinctive placement of the flash units tends to be at 9 and 3 o'clock simulating a 'ring flash' set-up (**Figures 56** and **57**). **Figures 58** to **69** show images with flash units in different positions.

The simple expedient of placing the flash units at 10 and 2 o'clock changes the impact of the highlights (**Figures 58** and **59**).

In the author's opinion, the Nikon clip on diffusers made a negligible difference to the highlights but improved the illumination of the buccal corridor (**Figures 62** and **63**).

Note the superior buccal corridor illumination when the lighting is on the same plane as the lens (see **Figure 69**).

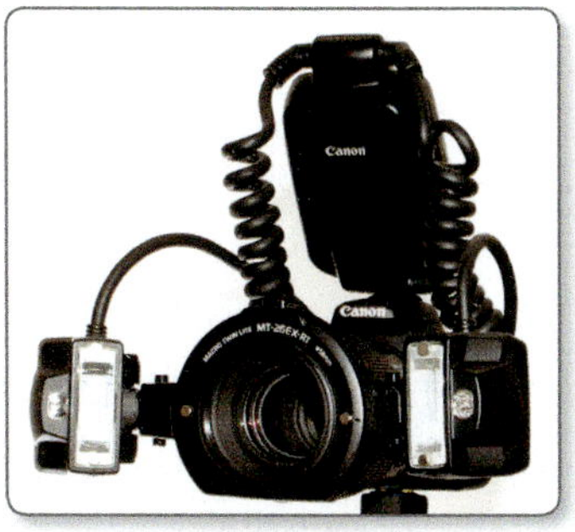

Figure 56 Canon MT 24/26 @ 9 and 3 o'clock on Canon mount.

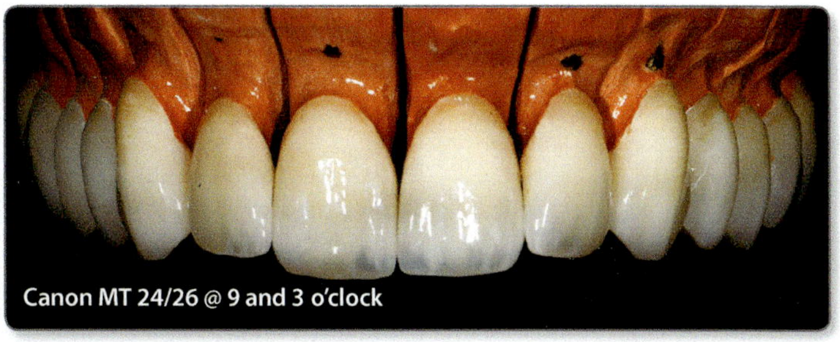

Figure 57 Image taken with MT 24 flash as shown in Figure 56.

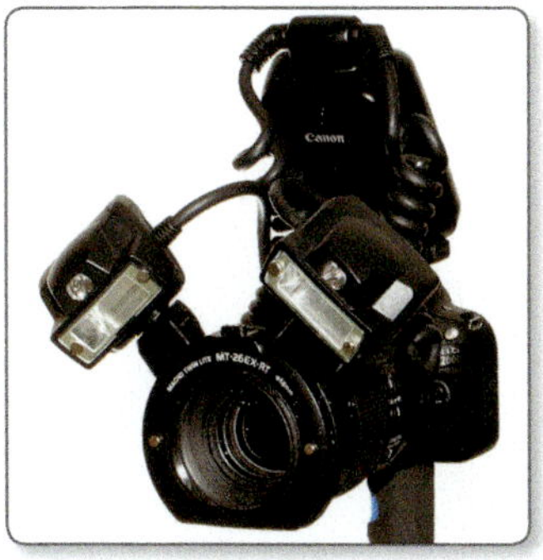

Figure 58 Canon MT 24/26 @ 10 and 2 o'clock on Canon mount.

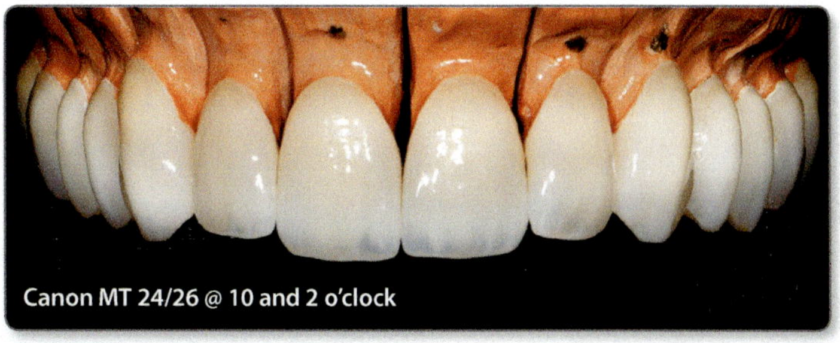

Figure 59 Image taken with MT 24 flash as shown in Figure 58.

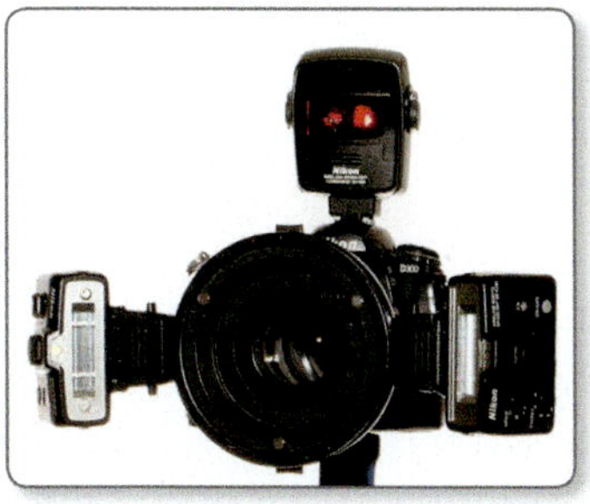

Figure 60 Nikon R1C1 flashes @ 9 and 3 o'clock on Nikon mount.

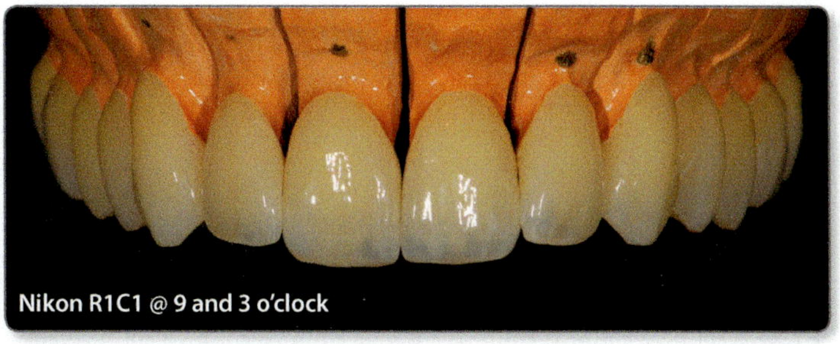

Figure 61 Image taken with R1C1 as shown in Figure 60.

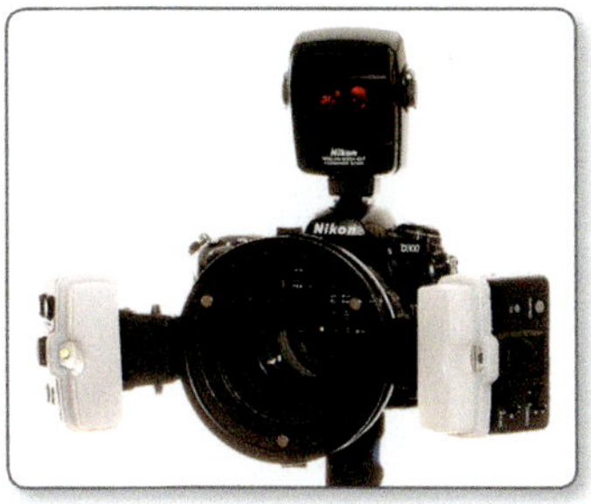

Figure 62 Nikon R1C1 flashes diffused.

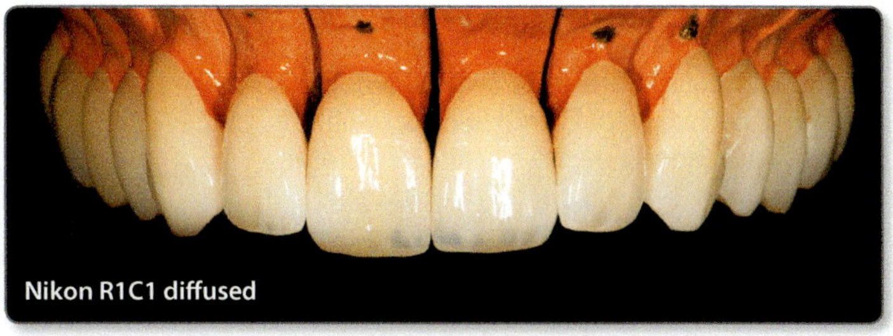

Figure 63 Image taken with R1C1 as shown in Figure 62.

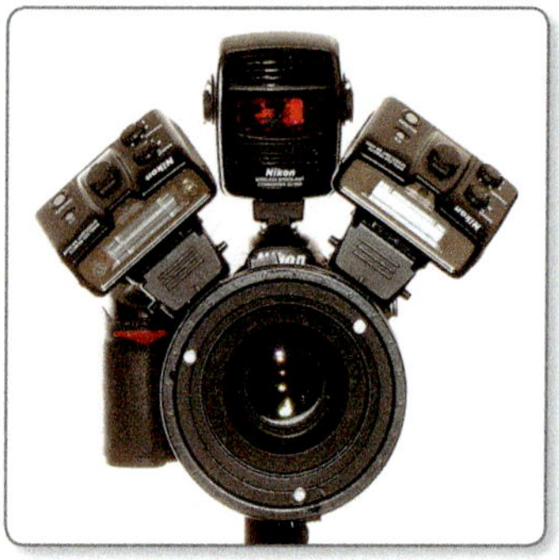

Figure 64 Nikon R1C1 flashes @ 10 and 2 o'clock.

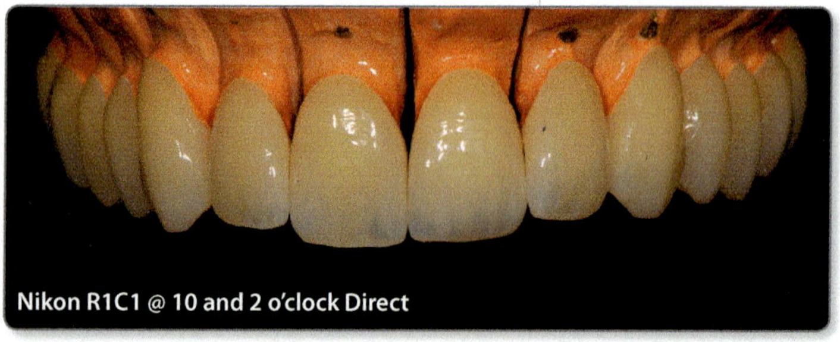

Figure 65 Image taken with R1C1 as shown in Figure 64.

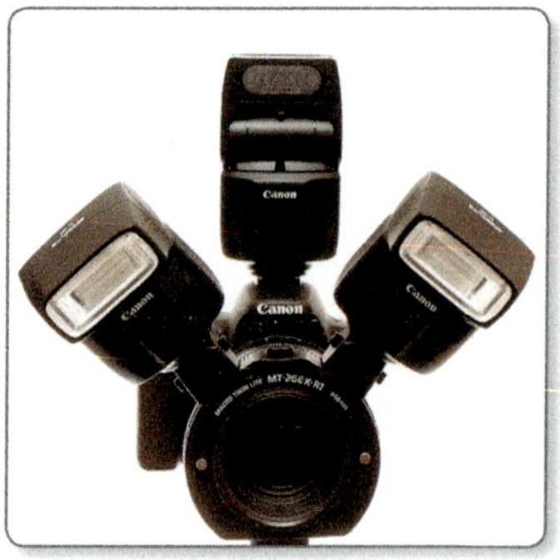

Figure 66 EL 100 flashes on MT 24/26 bracket.

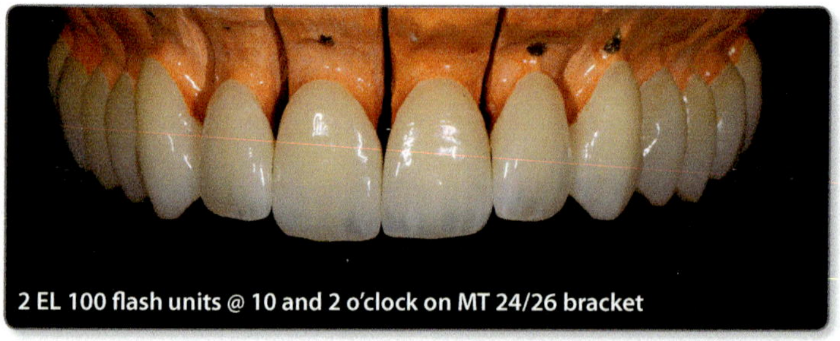

Figure 67 Image taken with set-up as shown in Figure 66.

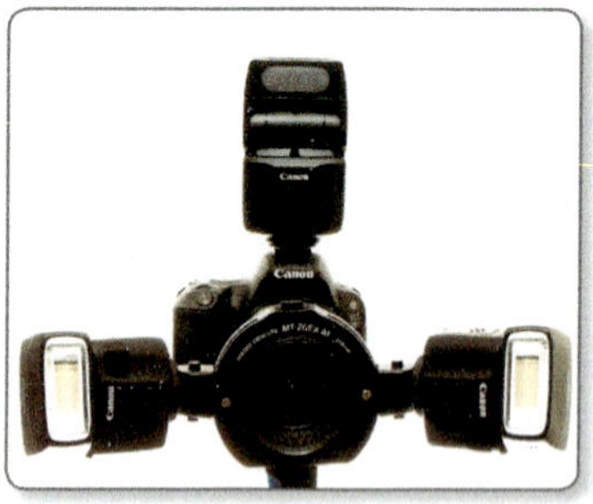

Figure 68 EL 100 flashes on MT 24/26 bracket.

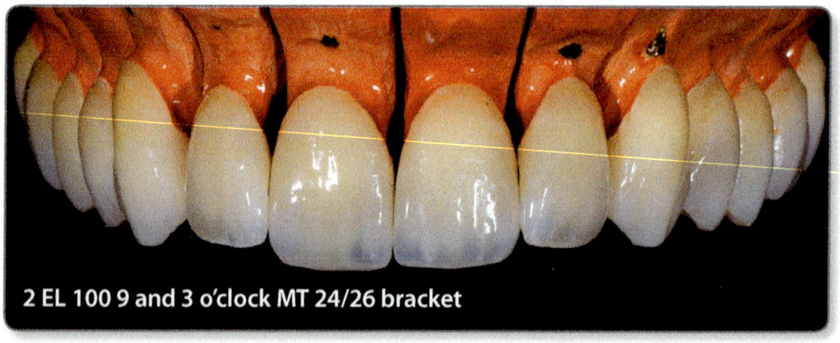

Figure 69 Image taken with EL 100 as shown in Figure 68.

All the previous images have been taken with direct flash and would be considered acceptable. It is obvious that moving the flash heads away from the subject reduces the impact of the highlights and raising them above the lens can accentuate incisal translucency. The user will have to decide which is the most appropriate system to suit their aims.

Perhaps the following could be considered apt.

An aesthetic photograph of teeth should have enough highlights to show vitality but not to obscure anomalies or pathology (**Figure 70**).

With the increasing demand for aesthetics and occasional reproduction of nature's flaws it has become more essential that illumination highlights do not obscure surface or sub-surface details.

Images of all shiny objects will have specular highlights which invariably enhance the subject, the object of this chapter is to investigate various lighting set-ups and compare results.

Bracket systems compared

Except for the Axis bracket all systems can offer an almost infinite variety of set-ups. Hopefully the examples shown in **Figures 71** to **78** will aid the reader.

Of the flash units tried on brackets, only the Canon MT 24/26 has the flash heads tethered to the power pack by a coiled lead. All the other flash systems were free standing and triggered wirelessly, and thus providing much lighter and more flexible combinations (**Figures 77** to **79**).

Soft boxes and bouncers

These accessories soften the lighting. Soft boxes work by spreading the area of the light source and reducing its intensity; bouncers are used to reflect the light from the flash source to produce indirect lighting. The most popular are produced by Lumiquest in the US but a new system has been introduced by Organic Dentistry in Portugal and described later in this chapter.

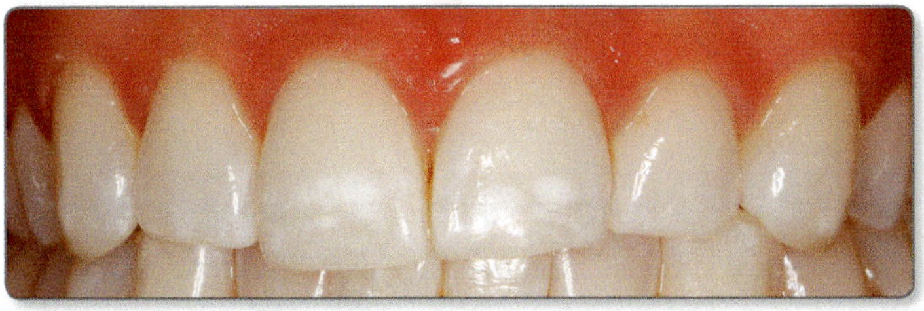

Figure 70 Image taken with Canon T24/26 system with minimal masking of pathology.

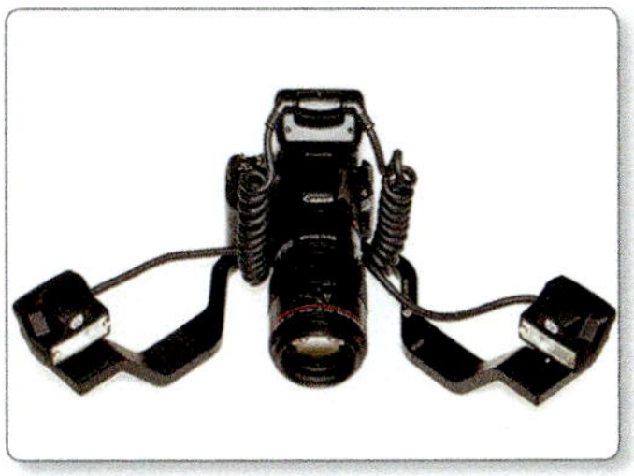

Figure 71 Canon MT 24/26 system on Axis bracket.

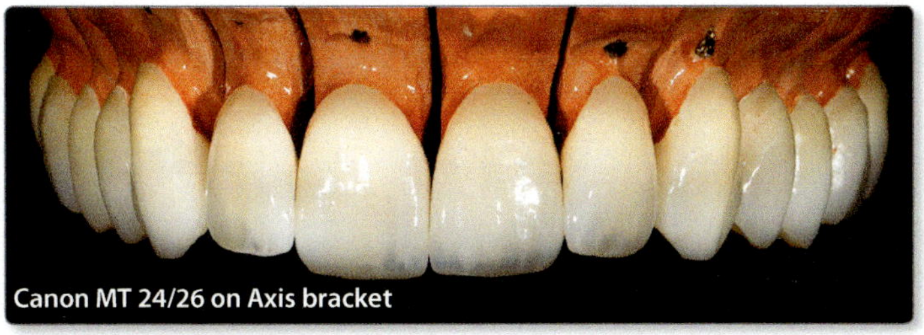

Figure 72 Image taken with set-up as shown in Figure 71.

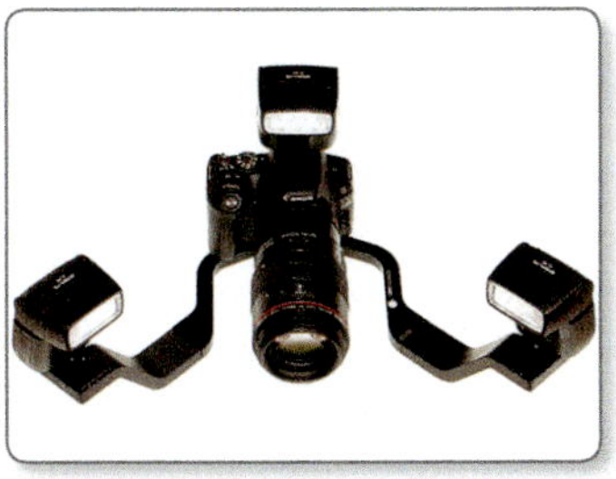

Figure 73 Canon EL 100 flashes on Axis bracket.

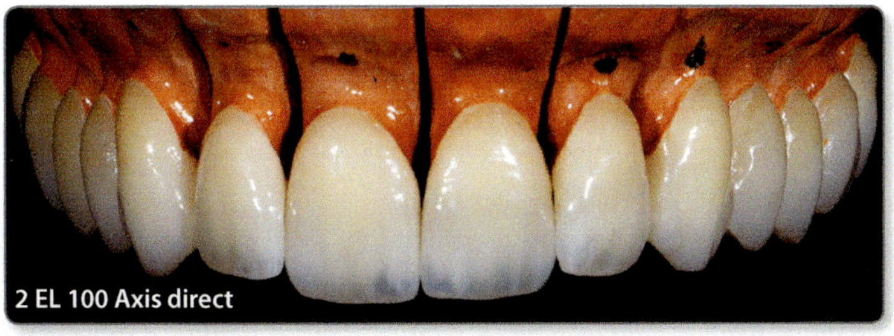

Figure 74 Image taken with set-up as shown in Figure 73.

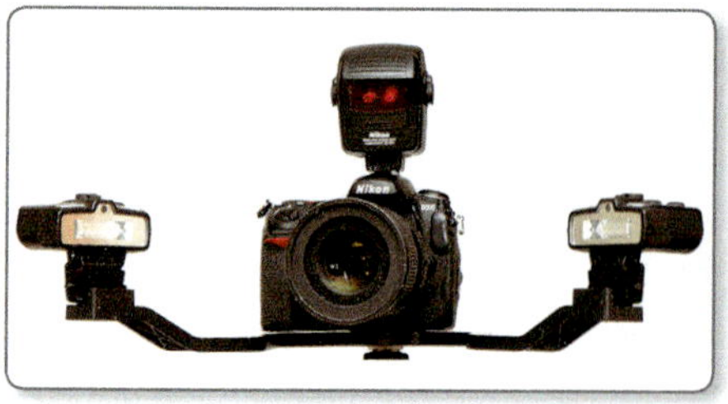

Figure 75 Nikon R1C1 system on Axis bracket.

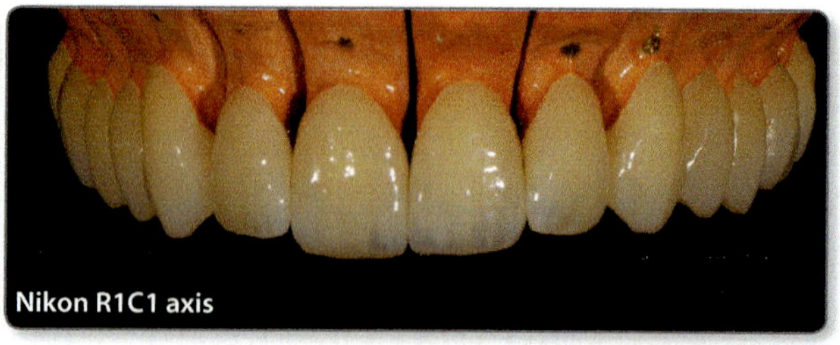

Figure 76 Image taken with set-up as shown in Figure 75.

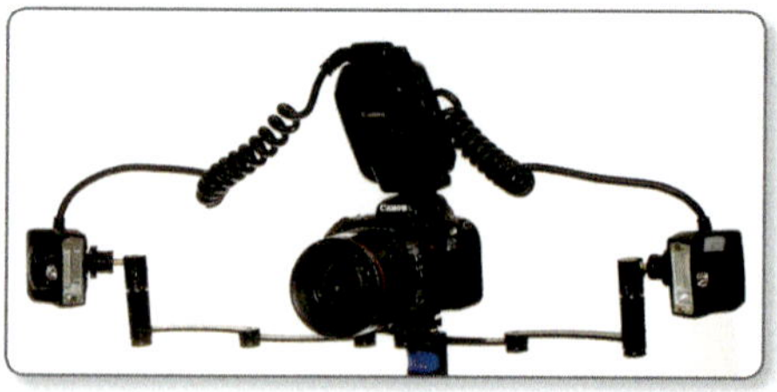

Figure 77 Canon MT 14/26 flash on Owl bracket extended.

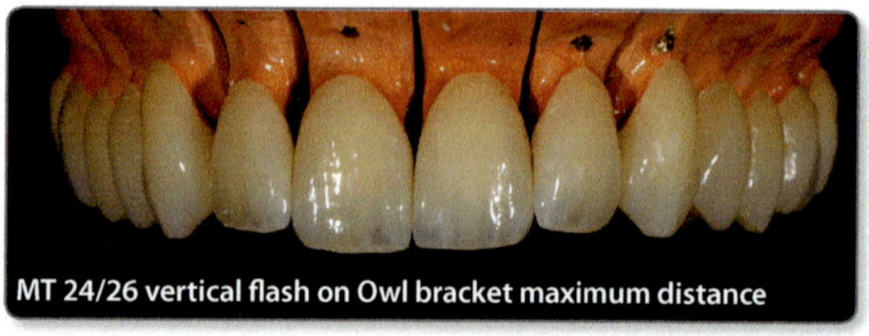

Figure 78 Image taken with set-up as shown in Figure 77.

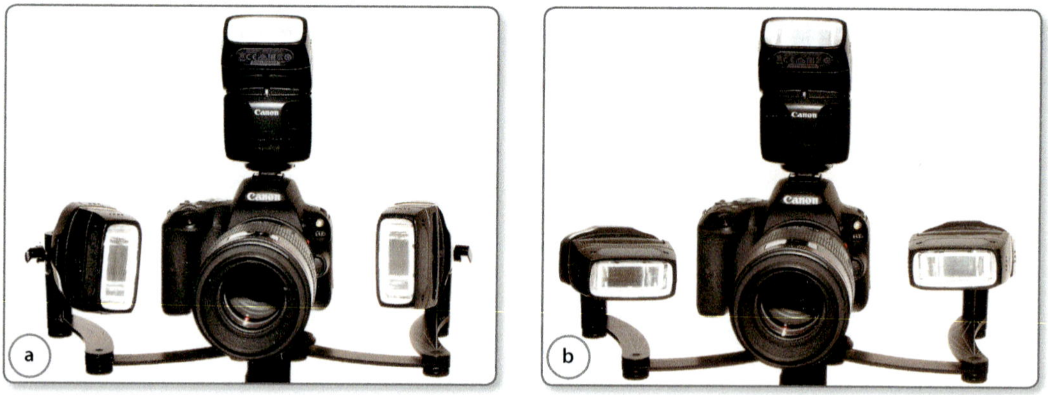

Figures 79a and b EL 100 flash units + third EL 100 as trigger for a wireless set-up on Owl bracket.

It is not practical to attach boxes or bouncers to either the small Nikon SB R200 or the Canon MT 24/26 flash heads, but the Canon EL 100 flash units can be fitted into the MT 24/36 mount and triggered wirelessly using a third EL 100 (see **Figure 68**).

Soft boxes are used on flashes facing the subject; bouncers reflect light from flashes facing away from the subject (see **Figures 80** to **82**).

To summarize, there is no right or wrong way to use soft boxes or bouncers for dental photography, it is a matter of experimentation and practice. Examples with various lighting set-ups are shown from **Figures 83 to 96**. There are pitfalls however and photography of static models differs from live patients. Whilst lighting from above can accentuate incisal translucency it can also increase shadow from the upper lips (see **Figure 90**).

One of the problems when using brackets and bouncers is the difficulty and practicality when switching from one type of photography to another and the possible need for an extra set-up. One solution is shown in **Figure 97**. An Axis bracket is shown with two Canon EL 100 flash units which easily accept soft boxes and bouncers. These two units are triggered wirelessly by the EL 100 flash in the hot shoe. A Metz MS-1 ring flash is mounted on the lens which is also triggered wirelessly by the EL 100 in the hot shoe. Changing from one lighting system to another is simply accomplished by turning on the appropriate flashes. Full Through The Lens (TTL) metering is maintained with this set-up which is considerably cheaper and more flexible than using flash systems with camera mounted power packs.

Obviously, this set-up is compatible with other bracket systems. The advantage of the Axis is that it is noticeably lighter in comparison with the others (see **Figure 97**).

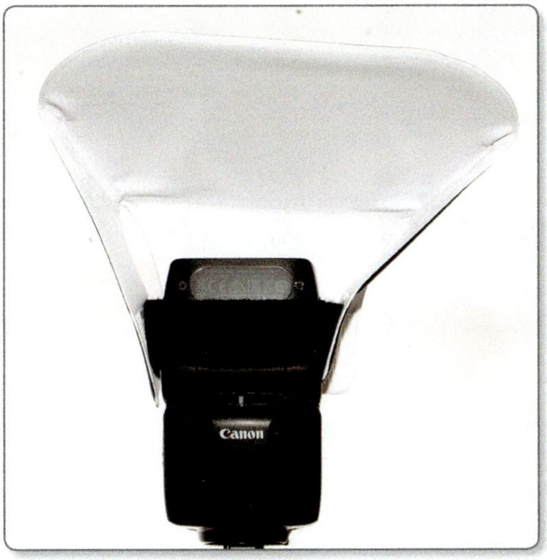

Figure 80 Lumiquest pocket bouncer.

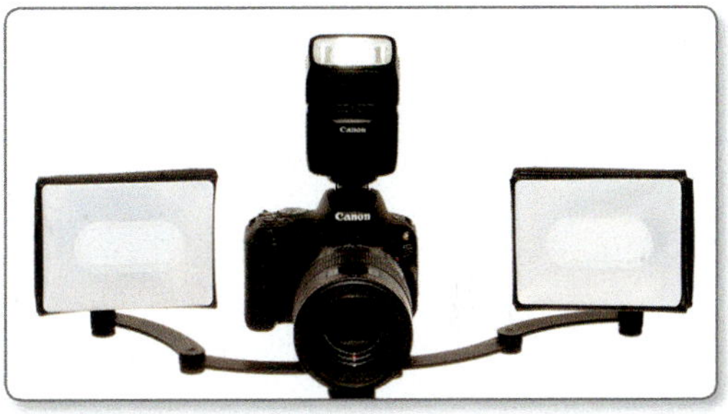

Figure 81 Lumiquest mini soft box.

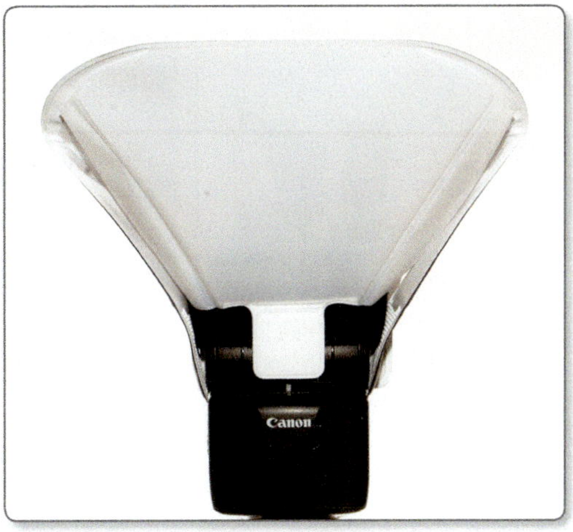

Figure 82 Lumiquest ultrasoft bouncer.

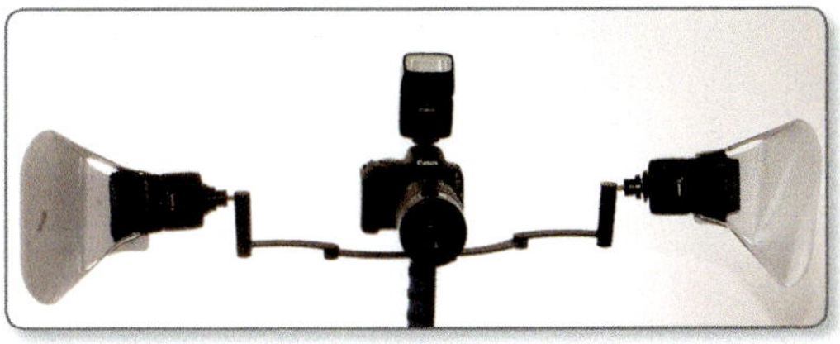

Figure 83 Two Canon EL 100 flash units on Owl bracket and Lumiquest bouncers.

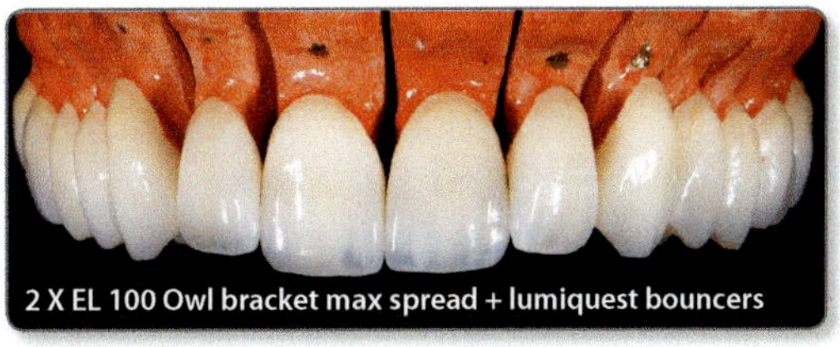

Figure 84 Two EL 100 + bouncers as shown in Figure 83.

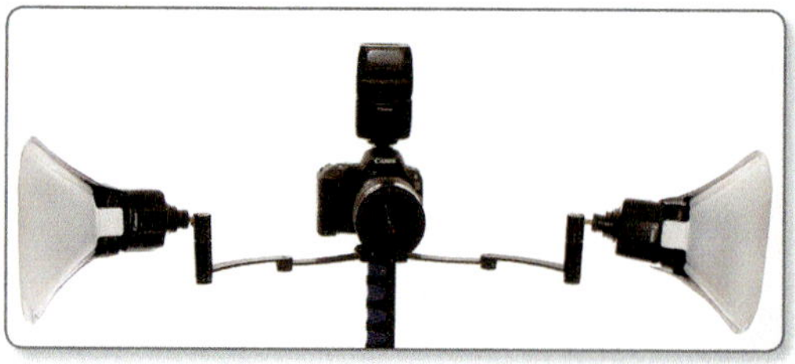

Figure 85 Two EL 100 flash + EL 100 as trigger + ultrasoft bouncers.

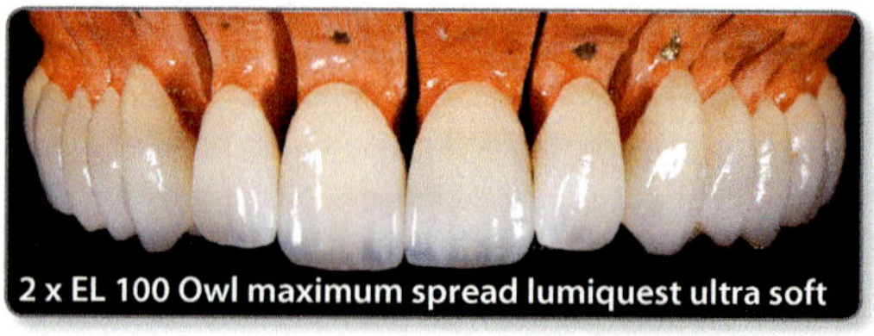

Figure 86 Image using set-up as shown in Figure 85.

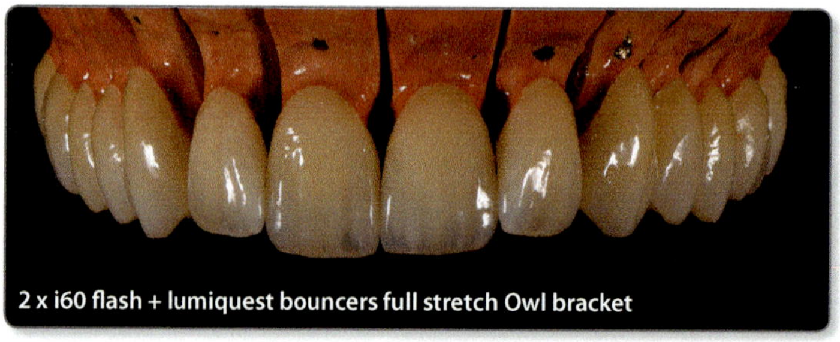

Figure 87 Image using 2 Nissin i60 flash units on Owl bracket as Figure 83.

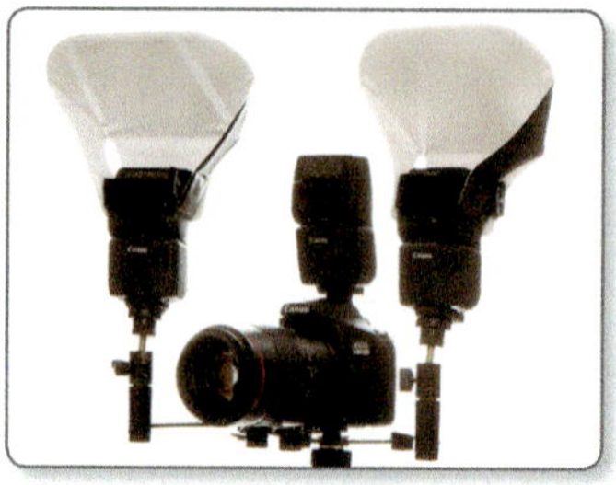

Figure 88 Lumiquest Bouncers above lens on Owl bracket.

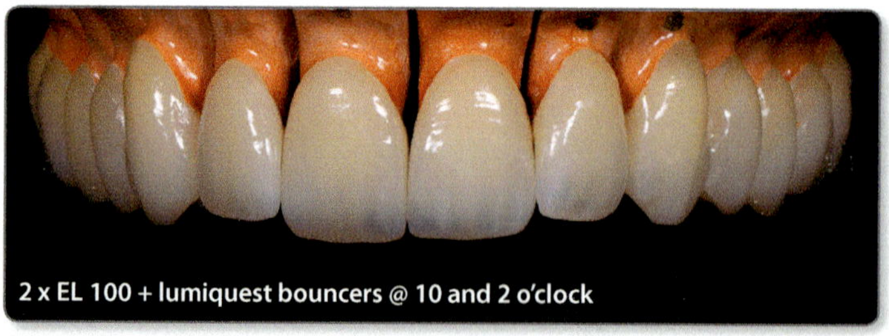

Figure 89 Image using set-up as shown in Figure 88.

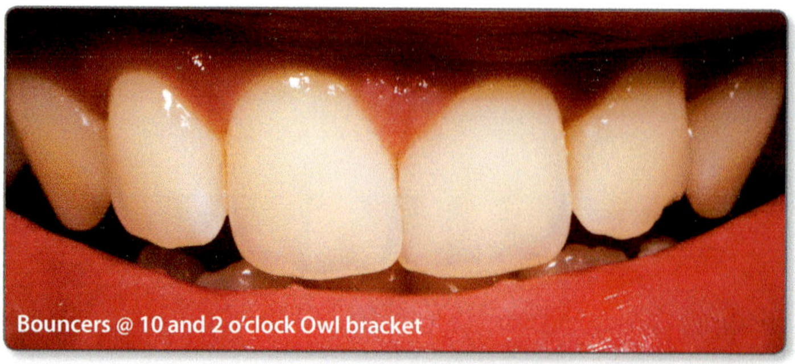

Figure 90 Image using set-up as shown in Figure 88 (note marked shadow from upper lip when light source is high).

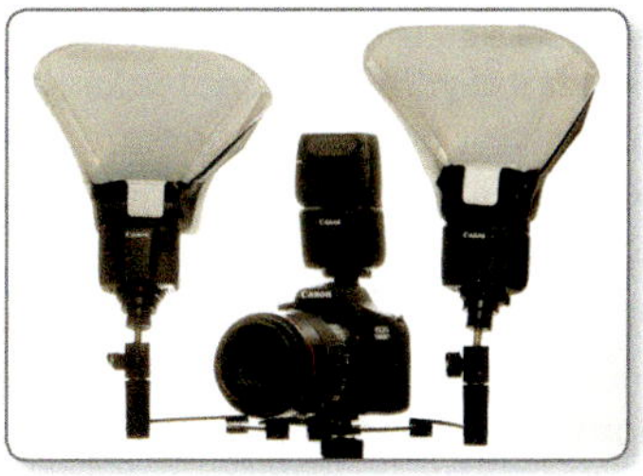

Figure 91 Lumiquest ultrasoft bouncers.

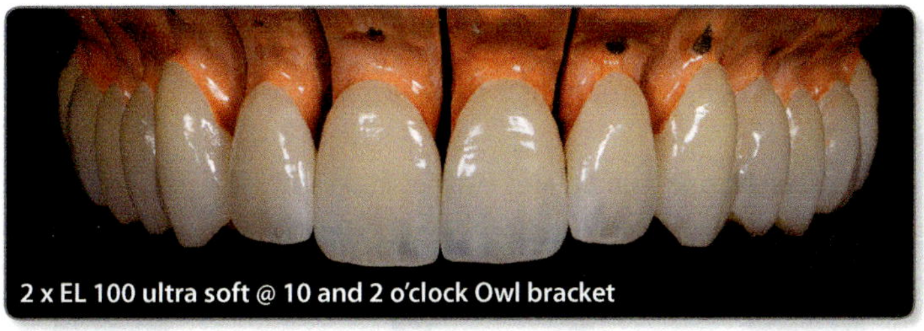

Figure 92 Image using set-up as shown in Figure 91.

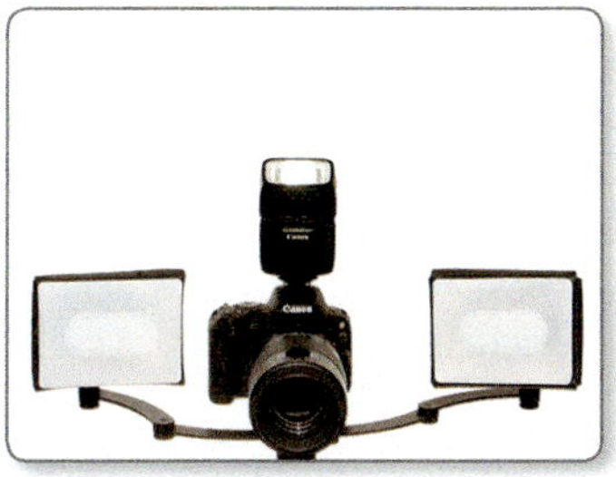

Figure 93 Nissin i60 flash units + mini soft boxes on Owl bracket 20 cm from lens.

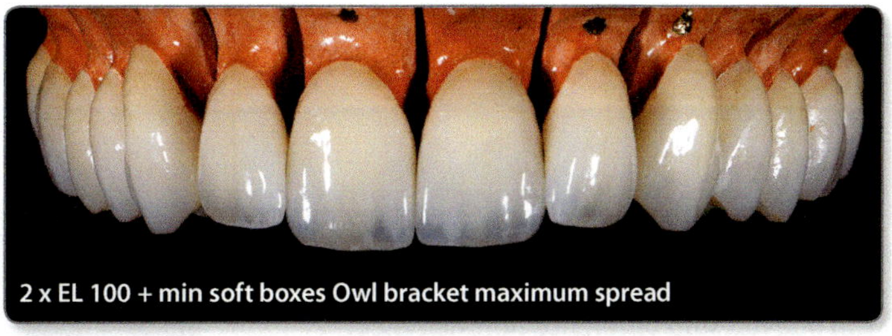

Figure 94 Image using set-up as shown in Figure 93.

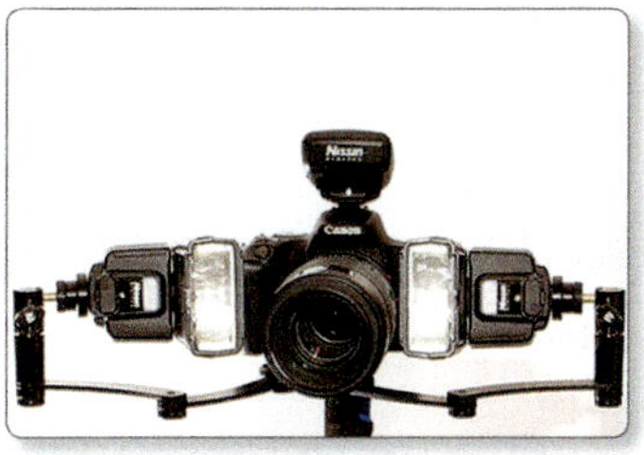

Figure 95 Two Nissin i60 flash units on Owl bracket + Nissin air trigger.

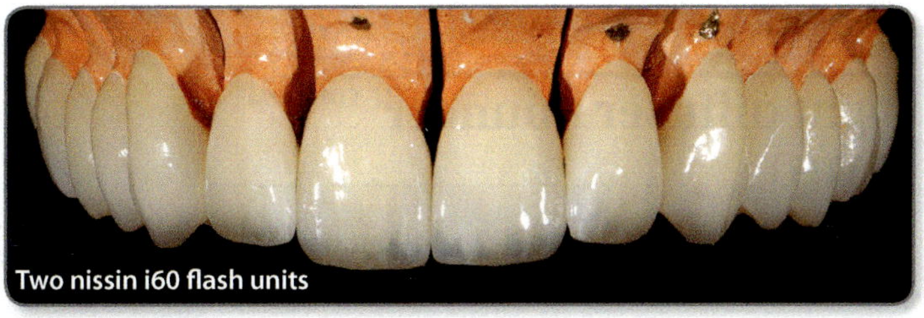

Figure 96 Image with set-up as shown in Figure 95.

Flash exposure bracketing

All current DSLR cameras offer the facility of varying their automatic exposure algorithms, the more expensive the camera, the greater the selection of the viewfinder area that can be chosen. For this reason, the author advises spot or centre-weighted metering as the best choice in general. There are often situations where the results are disappointing and either a darker or lighter image would have been preferable. This can be achieved with cameras offering a facility known as exposure bracketing and can be selected for ambient light photography. Depending on the camera, the operator chooses a degree of over and underexposure and takes a series of three or five images in quick succession. This results in one or two images brighter and darker than the automatically selected exposure, and the operator can make his or her choice of the best photograph.

The above facility is applicable to ambient light photography only, and is completely different to Flash Exposure Bracketing (FEB) which is available on fewer cameras or flash systems. The principle is as the above but in this

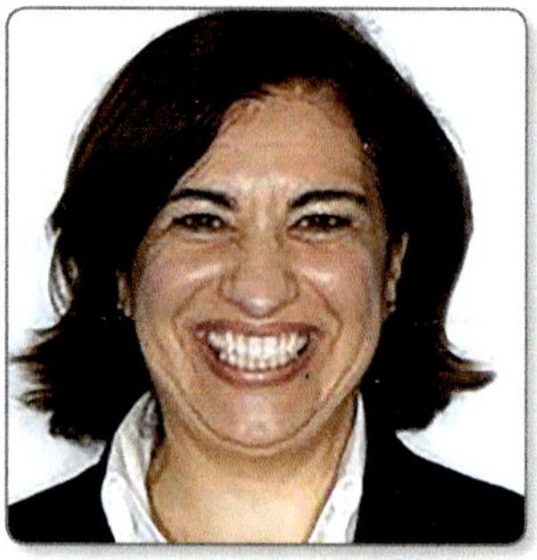

Figure 107 Full face using MT 24/26 flash with LDB etc. using setup Figure 103.
(*Courtesy:* Dr Hugo Lapa)

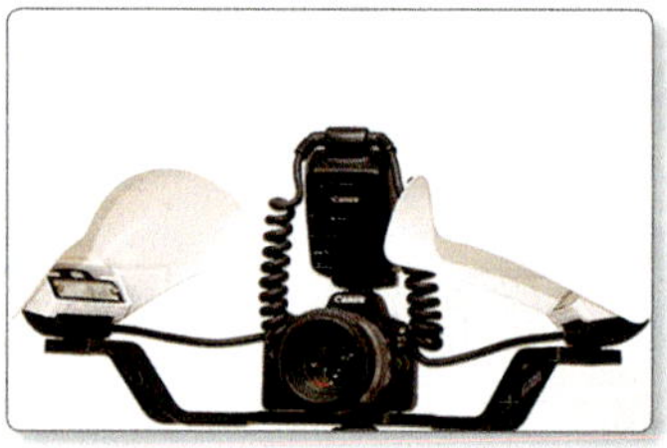

Figure 108 LDB on Axis bracket.

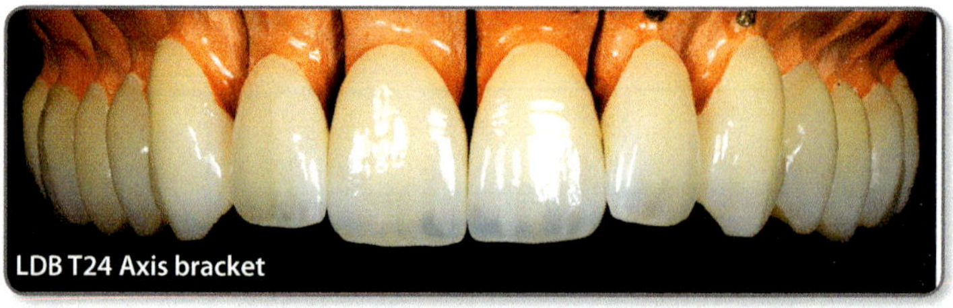

Figure 109 Image using set-up as Figure 108.

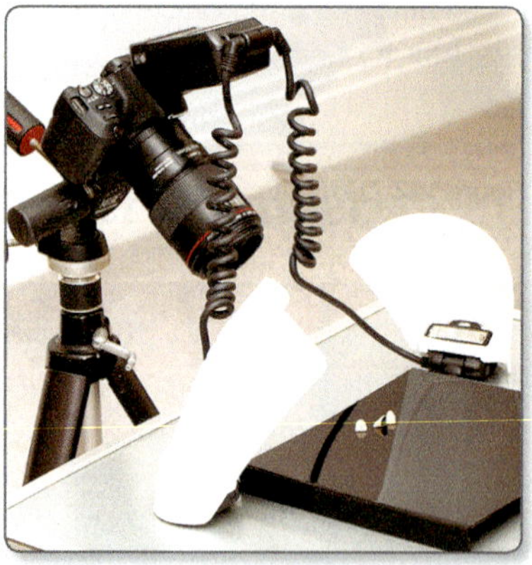

Figure 110 LDB's used as light tent.

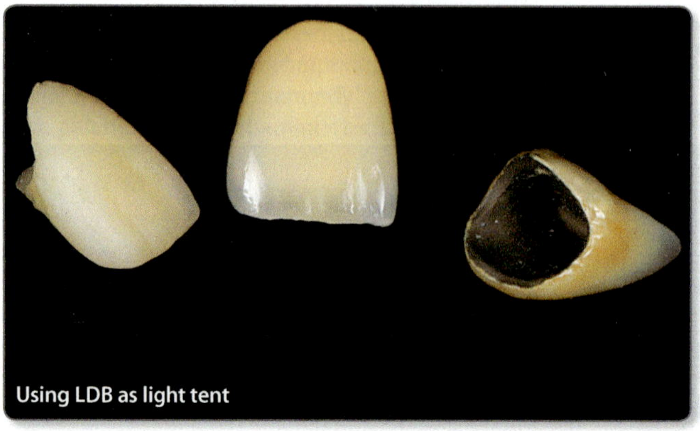

Figure 111 Image from Figure 110 set-up.

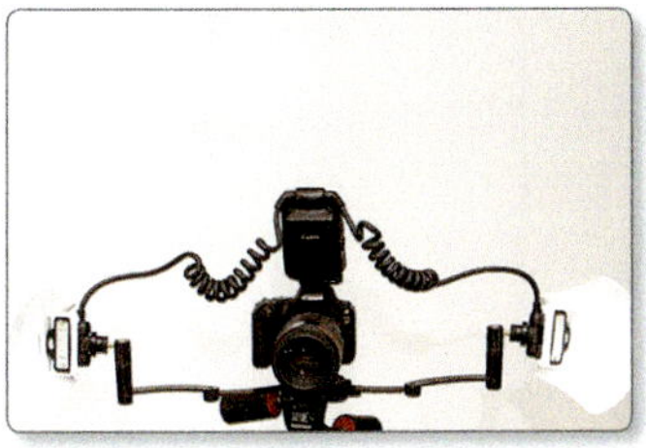

Figure 112 Set-up for Figure 113.

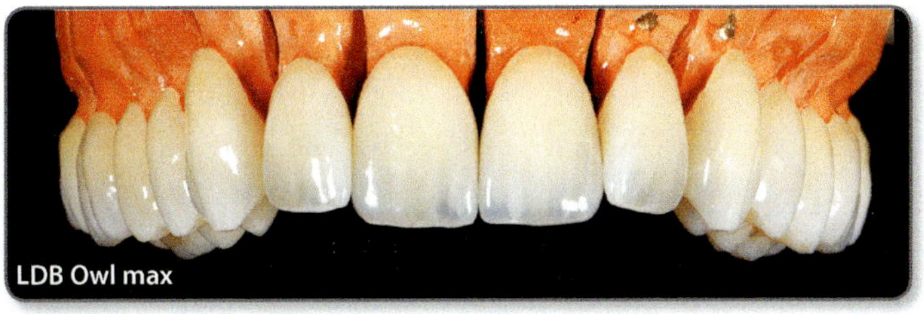

Figure 113 Image taken with flash units on Owl bracket as Figure 112.

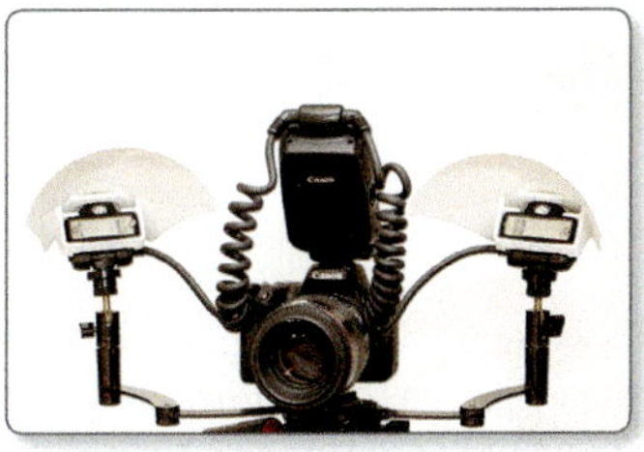

Figure 114 Set-up for Figure 115.

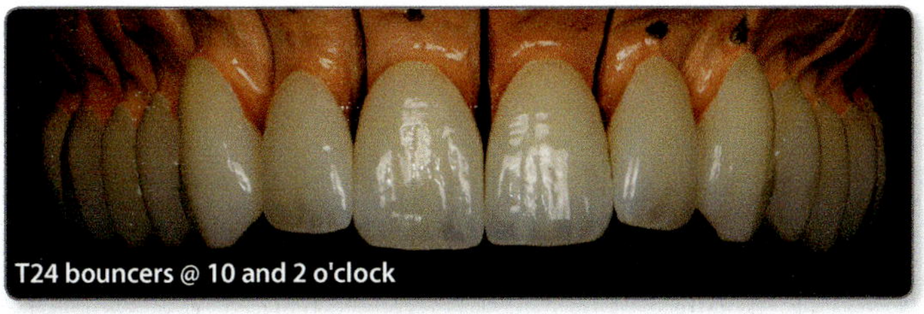

Figure 115 Image taken with set-up as Figure 114.

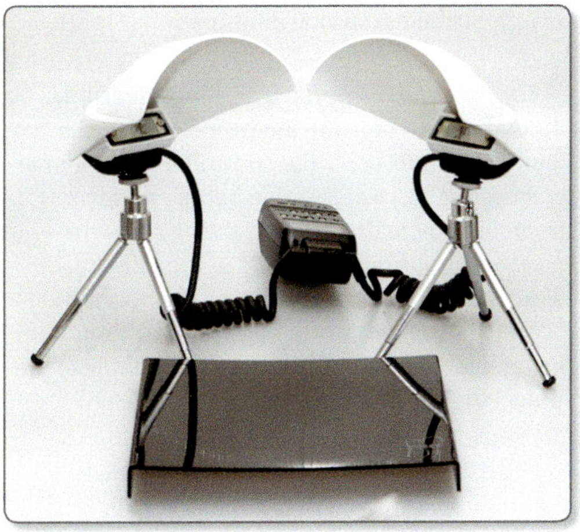

Figure 116 Set up using extension cord Figure 118.

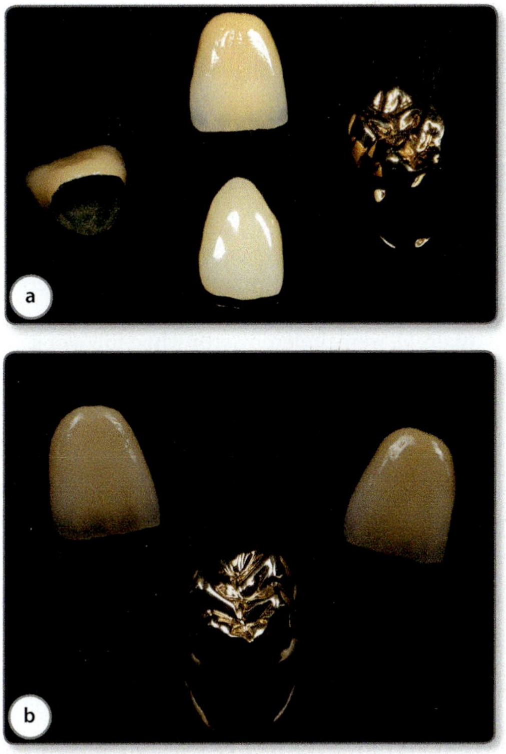

Figure 117 Image using set-up as Figure 116.

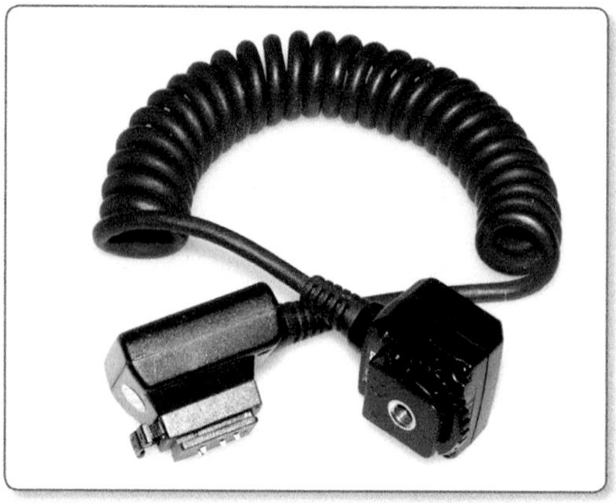

Figure 118 TTL extension cord.

Table-top photography

Whilst the author recommends "eye-level" focusing for virtually all clinical photography, using the rear screen to focus comes into its own in "table-top" photography. This involves putting the camera into "Live View" mode which is indicated by a button with a "camera" icon on Canon bodies and a small lever labeled "LV" on Nikon. The use of a good tripod is recommended for this type of photography.

Continuous lighting

Up to this point, the chapter has described various flash systems. The author has tried several budget LED continuous lighting systems, but virtually all were underpowered when following the mantra from film days of, "low ISO for quality + small aperture (f22) for depth of field." By increasing the ISO (sensitivity of the sensor) it is possible to achieve a compromise of a shutter speed high enough to avoid camera shake (1/125 second minimum) and a small aperture of f22. This topic is covered in greater detail in Chapter 4. If considering purchase of a continuous light source as covered here, the purchase of a "stabilised" lens would be considered essential.

Doctorseyes

The major advantage of continuous lighting is that focusing is greatly facilitated as the subject is fully illuminated. One continuous LED lighting system that can be considered for clinical photography is produced by "Doctorseyes."

The doctorseyes system uses a lens mount with magnets to hold the ring light (see **Figure 119**). Several mounts are available to cope with a range of lens filter mount sizes.

Two lighting systems are available, either a single ring **Figure 120** or with supplementary wing lights for additional illumination (**Figure 121).**

The lights are powered by a controller fitted under the camera using the tripod socket (see **Figures 122** and **125**). The controller incorporates an inaccessible rechargeable battery and has the facility to create various lighting scenarios by selecting various segments of the LEDs (see **Figure 125**). Continuous lighting is a boon when focussing intra orally but, in the author's opinion, the intensity of the lights is not comfortable to the subject for full face photography.

Figure 120 shows the ring light with the facility to attach the wing units. Doctorseyes also manufacture a slightly smaller ring light with without this facility together with a less sophisticated power-pack.

The author noticed that if both the wings and ring light were on at full power, the illumination of the buccal corridor was insufficient (see **Figure 123**).

However, by reducing the intensity of the ring light (see **Figure 124**), the overall exposure was more even.

The control buttons on the left change the arrays of the LEDs, which are displayed on the screen as shown in **Figure 126.**

From the above figures an ISO rating of 1600 would be considered suitable.

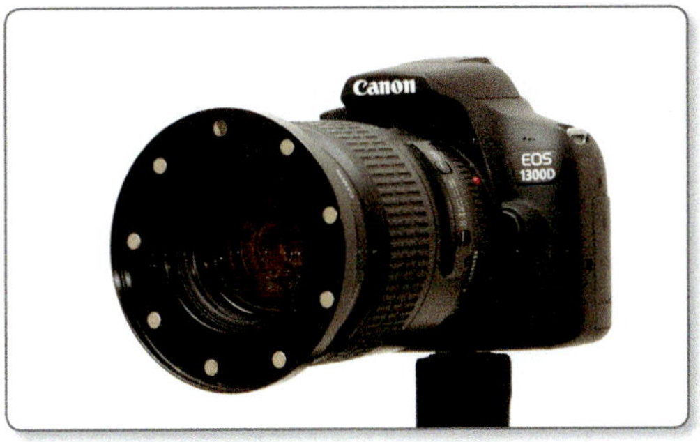

Figure 119 Magnetic lens mount.

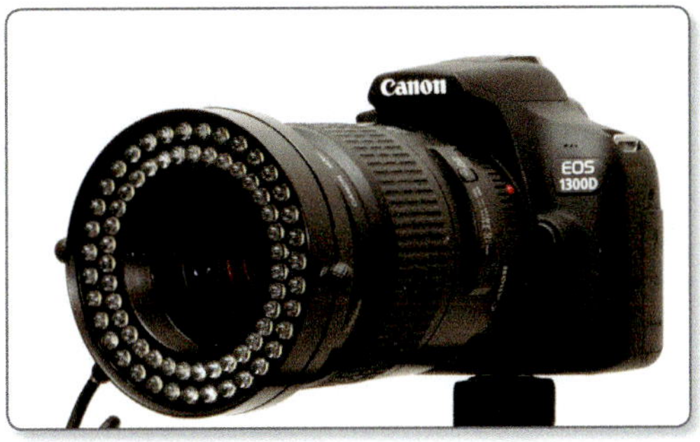

Figure 120 Ring light.

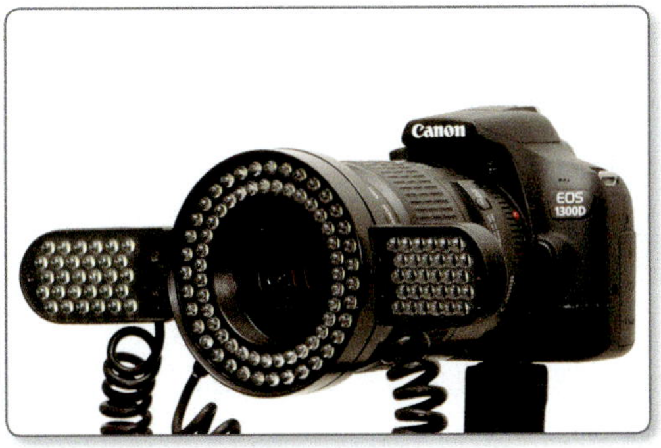

Figure 121 Ring light + wing lights.

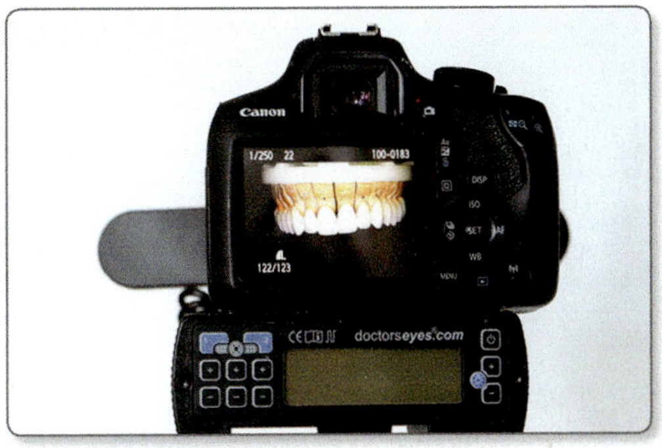

Figure 122 Camera with controller fitted.

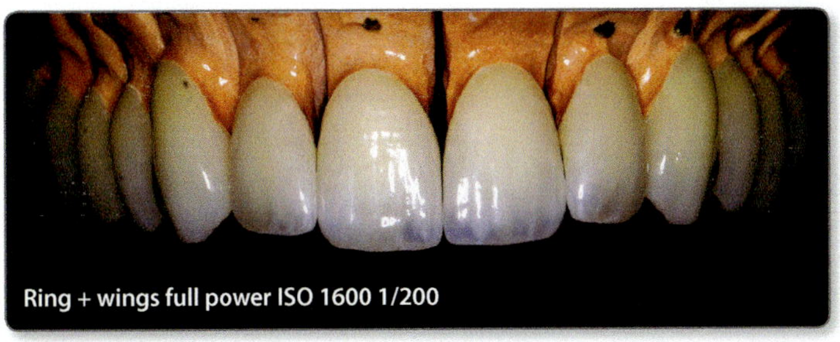

Figure 123 Ring light and wing lights at full power.

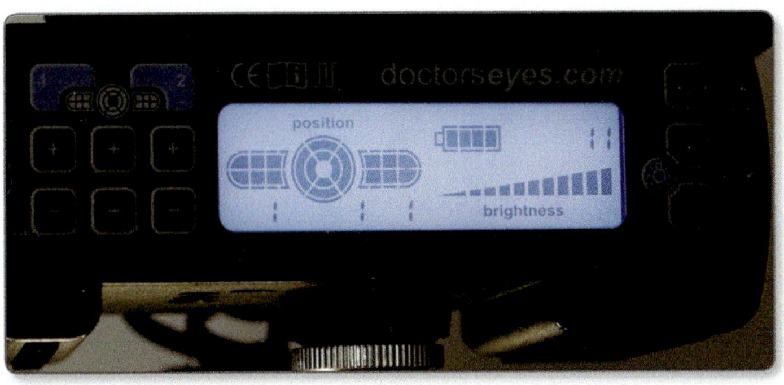

Figure 124 Control unit. Doctorseyes power pack showing ring and wing lights at full power.

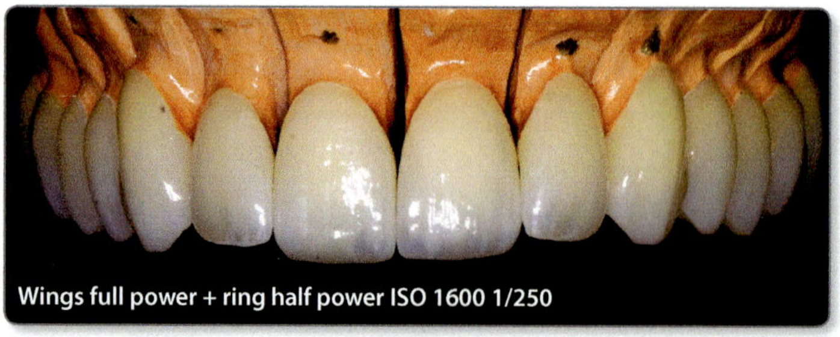

Figure 125 Image using wing lights at full and ring light at half power.

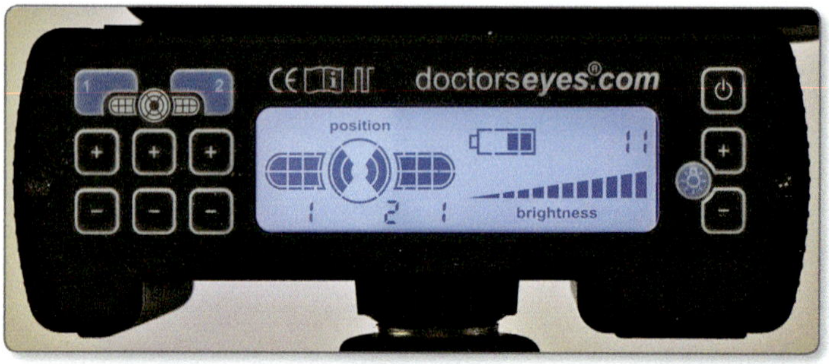

Figure 126 Control unit. Doctorseyes powerpack showing wing lights at full power and ring light at half power.

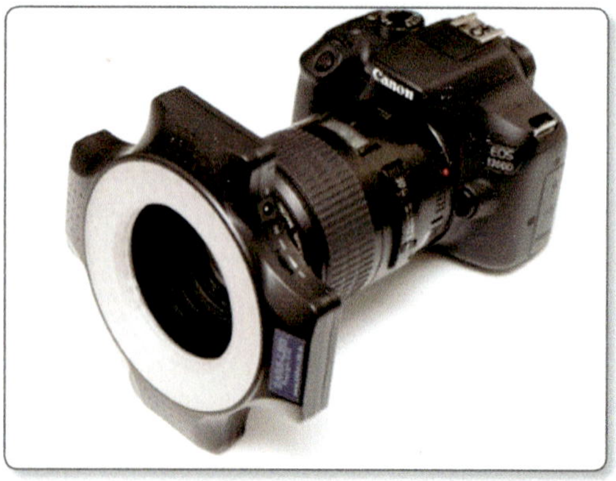

Figure 127 SARA-LED 60 .

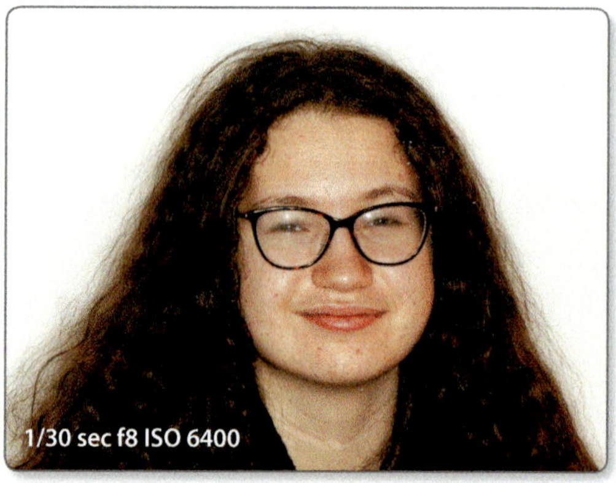

Figure 128 Image taken using SARA-LED 60.

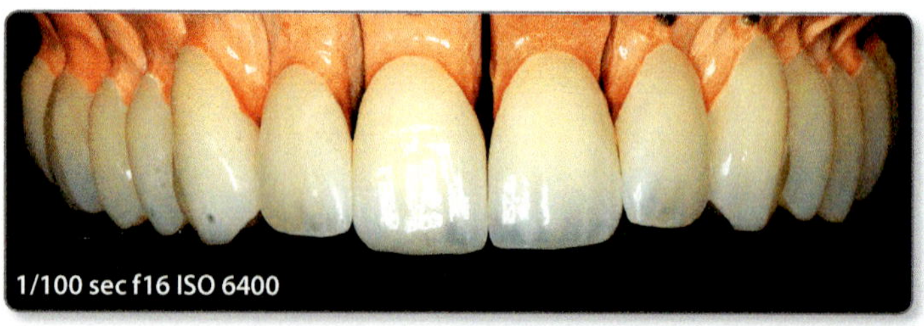

Figure 129 Image taken using SARA-LED 60 .

SARA-LED 60

One other “lower power” LED system used by the author is the SARA-LED 60 (**Figure 127**). As the name suggests it has 60 LEDs as the light source and powered by four AA cells mounted around the light.

The SARA-LED 60 is considerably less powerful than the doctorseyes system and the author found that an ISO of 6400 was required to attain satisfactory images. At portrait distance the aperture had to be increased to f8 to allow a reasonable shutter speed of 1/30 which is not ideal when using 100 mm lens (see **Figure 128**).

Even using an ISO of 6400 required an aperture of f16 to allow a shutter speed of 1/100 second (see **Figure 129**).

4 Setting up a DSLR for clinical use

Introduction

Dental photography with digital cameras can virtually be approached in at least two ways (see **Figure 1**):

- Firstly, and most commonly, is to follow all the advice given for film cameras and simply transfer it to a digital body. 'Dental Photography' by Wander & Gordon; Br Dent J. 1987
- Secondly, is to consider the advantages of modern technology and how to use them

The following recommendations are based on the author's 50 years of experience. They are not, 'set in stone' but have been found practical and successful and will work with all marques.

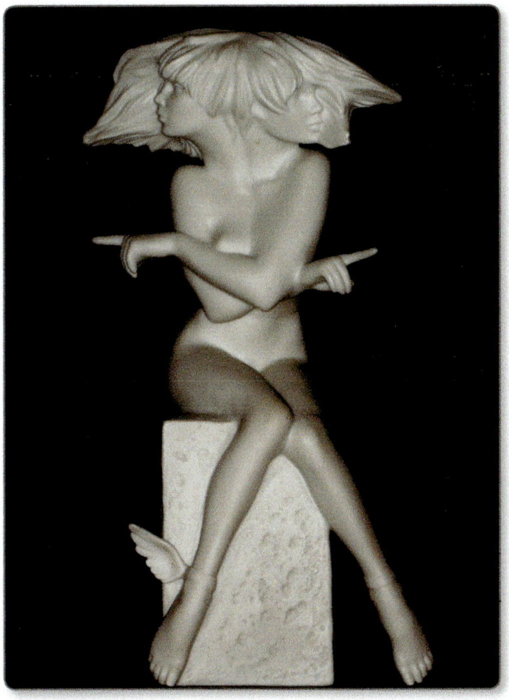

Figure 1 'Gemini' (Royal Copenhagen).

The reasoning behind this chapter is to preset the variables so that camera operation in the surgery is virtually little more than switching it on and off.

For those familiar with camera settings and terminology the protocol is summarised at this point with the explanation to follow.

It is assumed that the camera battery has been charged and the basic settings of date and time have been entered, if not, set them first. Apart from the 'Mode' setting, all the other presets will involve using the camera's menu. Remember that all manuals are available as free downloads, if required.

Camera body

Based on a 'transfer from film' policy, preset the following into the digital body.

- Disable the ability for camera to take images without a memory card in position
- Select an ISO sensitivity of 100 or 200
- Select the highest image quality
- Select, 'Hold' for the image review period or choose the longest review time available
- Select the metering area to centre weighted average or spot
- Set 'manual focus' (MF) on the lens and body, if appropriate
- Select aperture priority mode 'A' Nikon or 'AV' Canon
- Disable 'Red-Eye' function*
- Set white balance (WB) to electronic flash (Lightning icon ⚡)
- CANON select flash synchronisation speed in AV mode (see below)

* The reason for disabling the "RED EYE" function is as follows:- When enabled, the flash system fires a "pre-flash" causing pupils to contract and thus reduce the incidence of "RED EYE." Unfortunately the pre-flash cannot detect whether faces or teeth are being photographed so disabling the function is the best option.

Flash system

- Use the Mode button to select E-TTL for Canon, through-the-lens (TTL), or TTL-BL for Nikon to allow fully automatic flash illumination. (See the information window on the flash powerpack)
- Confirm the flash output of each tube is 1:1

If the camera and flash are set up as above, the only physical change of setting required is the aperture, from 'f8' for all full facial views to 'f22' for all oral and peri-oral views.

Multi-user situation

If there are several users of one camera even the simple change of aperture as above can be forgotten. For example, a face shot at f22 comes out underexposed, the operator forgets the simple aperture change, and makes other alterations to the settings which in turn causes problems for subsequent users. By making use of 'Modern Camera Technology' it is theoretically possible to set the ISO to 'Auto' and maintain an aperture of f22 throughout. The computer within the camera will automatically adjust the sensor sensitivity to achieve a correct exposure.

Unfortunately, this is not a universal facility which will be explained later in the text.

However, there is another option where one fixed aperture setting of f22 will work whatever the combination of camera and flash system. This involves setting the ISO to a higher level "permanently" which will allow full face images taken at about 2 metres distance to be correctly exposed using a standard ring-flash. Technically this lowers the quality of the final image but from the author's experience, modern sensors are so good, that even cropping a single molar from a full arch view is of publishing standard (see **Figures 2a** and **b**). Even with a high ISO of 1600 a single molar can be cropped satisfactorily (see **Figures 3a** and **b**).

From the sequence as shown in **Figures 4a** to **d** satisfactory exposures were attained at ISO's 6400, 3200, and 1600 and the exposure at ISO 800 was underexposed. Thus, selecting an ISO of 1600 together with the highest quality image, will allow satisfactory results with a permanent aperture setting of f22.

Similarly, maintaining a high ISO for the clinical shots the automatic exposure flash system works admirably. The following series of images demonstrate the quality of images at higher settings (**Figure 5**).

Modes

These options were described earlier in the book but will be expanded here as they lead to most of the issues between teachers on this subject. The choice of 'Mode' for dental photography is either 'M' manual, where the operator selects both the aperture and shutter speed, or 'A' (Nikon) 'AV' (Canon) aperture priority,

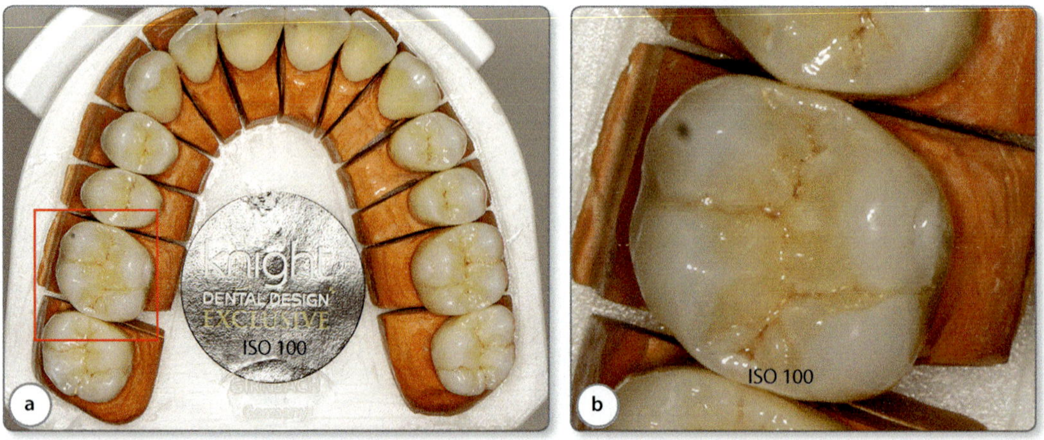

Figure 2 Images taken with an ISO setting of 100. (a) Shows a full arch, and (b) cropped molar enlarged from full arch image left.

where the operator selects the aperture and the camera automatically selects the shutter speed for the ambient conditions. However, in dental photography using electronic flash, the situation becomes slightly complicated because of the differing methods of flash operation between Canon and Nikon. As aperture controls the 'depth of field,' the author recommends the camera to be set in aperture priority mode. Using this set-up, the operator only needs to change apertures between full face and intra-/peri-oral views. TTL flash metering will automatically compensate for the changes both in aperture and subject to camera distance.

Either way, it is essential that other basic settings are made first.

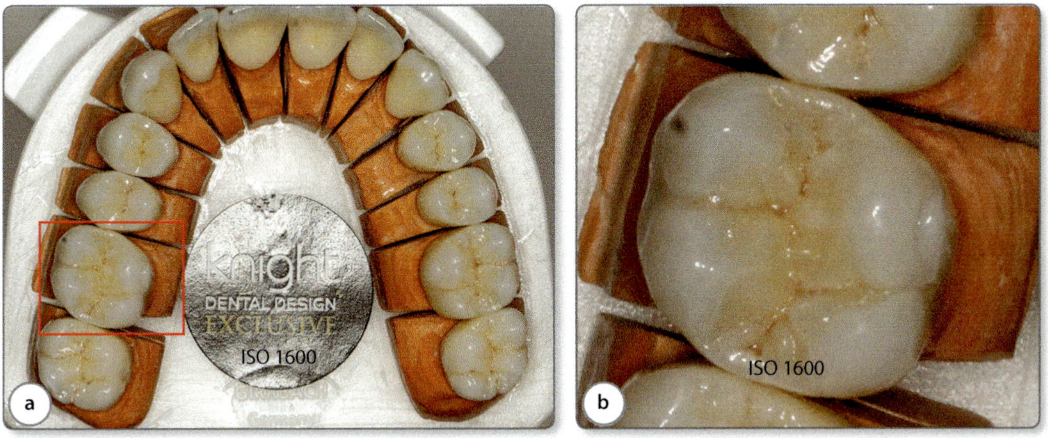

Figure 3 Images taken with an ISO setting of 1600. (a) Show the same arch, and (b) cropped molar enlarged from full image left.

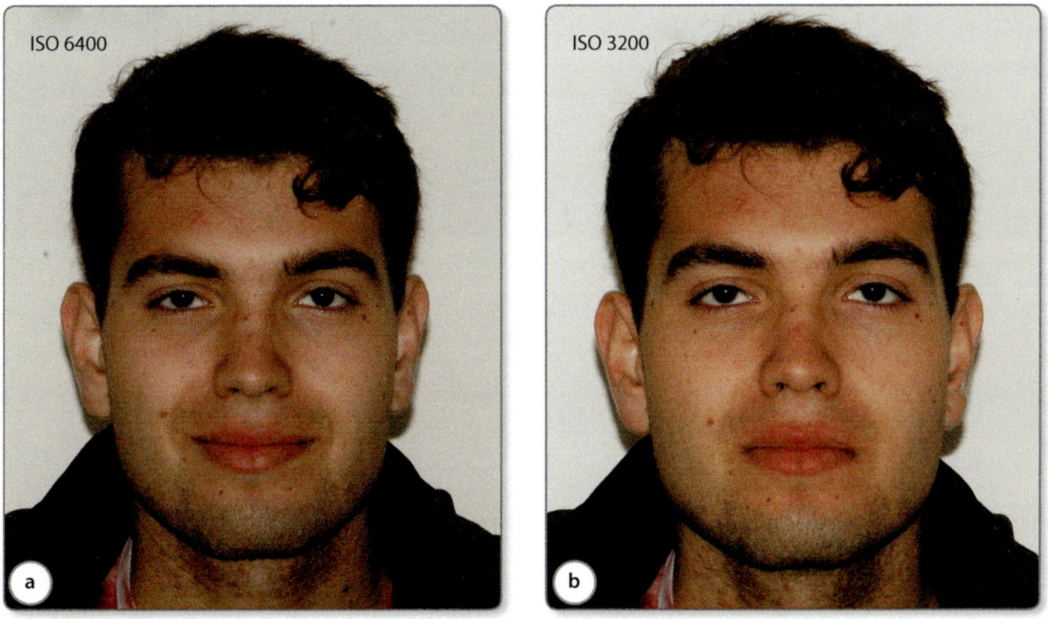

Figure 4 Facial views with a permanent aperture setting of f22 (a) ISO 6400; (b) ISO 3200; (c) ISO 1600; (d) ISO 800. *Continues overleaf*

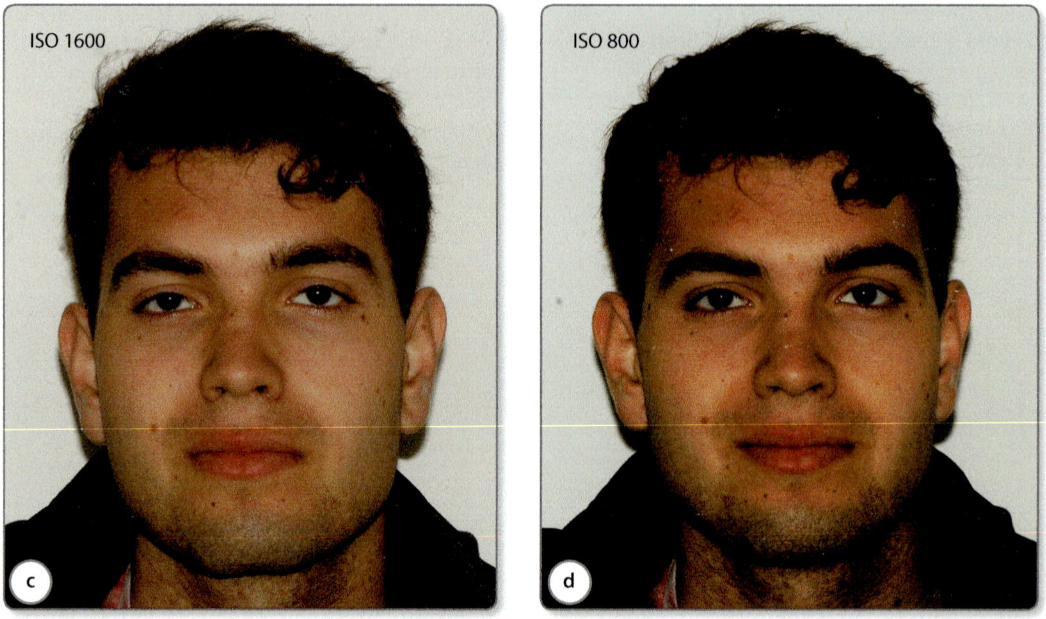

Figure 4 *Continued.*

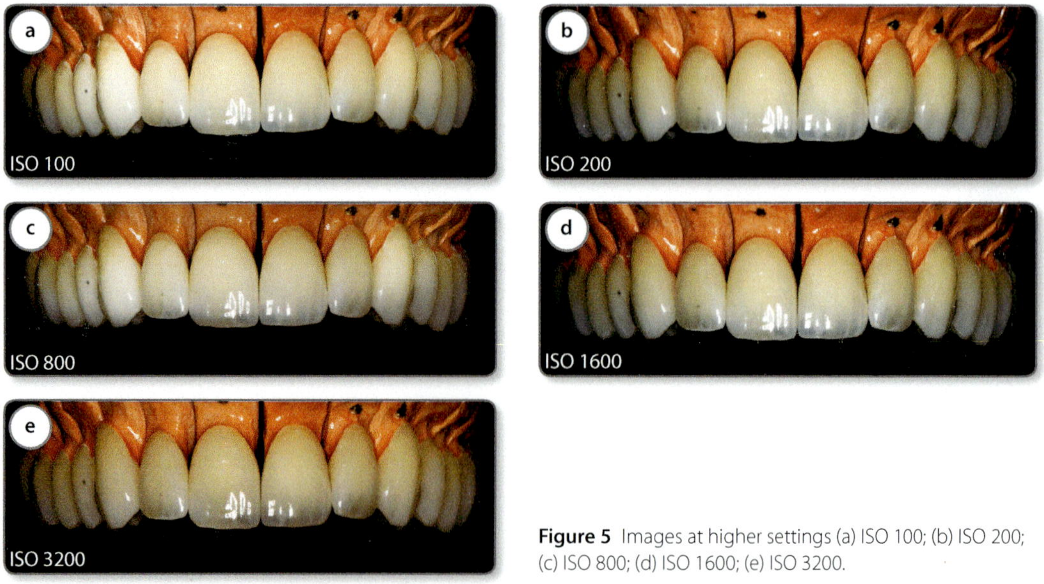

Figure 5 Images at higher settings (a) ISO 100; (b) ISO 200; (c) ISO 800; (d) ISO 1600; (e) ISO 3200.

Flash synchronisation speed

This was mentioned in Chapter 1 and is the recommended shutter speed when using electronic flash. It refers to a speed when the focal plane shutter is fully open for the extremely brief period of the flash.

Nikon

If 'A' aperture priority is set into a Nikon body and a flash unit is attached and switched 'ON' the shutter speed will default to the flash synchronisation shutter speed of 1/60 seconds automatically and aperture changes are made simply.

Canon

When 'M' manual mode is selected on most basic Canon cameras, the only operating wheel will change the shutter speed. If this is preset to 1/200 or 1/250 seconds for flash use, the +/– button must be depressed simultaneously with the thumb to enable the operating wheel to change the aperture only.

If 'AV' aperture priority is set into a Canon body, there is no default to the flash synchronisation speed of 1/200 or 1/250 seconds and certainly on the more basic models the only operating wheel changes the shutter speed as above. The solution is to preset the flash synchronisation speed in 'AV' mode via the camera's menu. The method can differ from model-to-model. On some models it is set under the 'Flash Control' menu, on others it is under 'Custom Functions.' Once this is set, only the aperture will change when using the operating wheel.

Aperture setting

Most clinical photography will be close-up where depth of field is paramount and an aperture of f22 is the one of choice. As the specialised flash systems for close-up photography are not as powerful as other general flash units, any facial views taken at f22 from approximately 2 metres, will be underexposed. Based on a direct transfer from film to digital and with the above presets, the aperture will need to be increased to f8. In summary, therefore, cameras set-up as above will require an aperture change from f22 intra- and peri-oral to f8 for faces. Generally, this simple change does not cause a problem. In the multi-user situation, especially orthodontic practices, difficulties often arise, as discussed earlier.

Modern technology

The choice of ISO sensitivity settings on many later camera bodies includes 'Auto' where the camera will automatically select the sensitivity to the duration and intensity of the illumination. Therefore, theoretically one can preset 'Auto' into the ISO setting and f22 on the aperture and use the system without any changes from close-ups to full faces. In practice, however, it is not necessarily so! Compatibility was discussed in Chapter 3 and certainly to guarantee full satisfactory operation with an ISO setting of 'Auto' the author recommends that at least the flash and camera are the same make. If using existing equipment with either matching or with third party accessories it would be a matter of trial and error. If new purchases are considered, then trying before buying would be greatly recommended.

Setting image quality

The author generally recommends setting the highest quality image 'L' as this will allow publication, if required. However as shown earlier in the chapter higher ISO values can be totally satisfactory.

Figure 6 shows the choice available on most cameras.

Audit trail

It may arise that the authenticity of a digital image is required. Pre-digital, in the UK the Crown Prosecution Service (CPS) would accept without question, a Polaroid image, a transparency, or print if the negative was available. Today, digital images are not necessarily that easy to authenticate. It is up to the reader to decide what

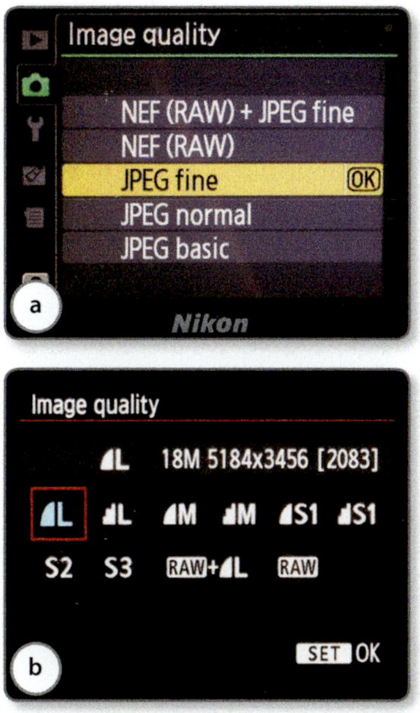

Figure 6 Typical choice of image quality.

level of security is needed, and perhaps select a higher level in certain circumstances.

Generally, the camera should be set up to give a high-quality image. This image will be processed within the camera and is the one that is seen on the screen at the back of the camera. This is colloquially known as a 'JPEG' (Joint Photographic Experts Group) image.

These images can be transferred to the patient's notes and would be available for any use later; however, they can also be easily manipulated.

Correspondence from 'Dental Protection Ltd.' suggests that a signed letter from the dentist that their image was accurate would suffice in most issues, on the 'basis of probability.' Minor changes such as straightening or cropping are accepted without an issue.

However, there may be situations where the photographic evidence must be, 'beyond reasonable doubt.' This can only be achieved in digital photography if the original image was also taken and available in what is known as RAW format. Currently in the UK there is a move to replace, "beyond reasonable doubt" with "satisfied so that you are sure."

A RAW image is the equivalent of a digital negative and can be compared with an exposed but unprocessed radiograph. The digital image is not processed within the camera but is processed by software in a computer later. By selecting RAW + L in the set-up menu, the camera will automatically record two images, one in RAW format, the other as a high-quality JPEG. The author suggests transferring the JPEG image to the patient's notes and keeping the RAW images on a separate hard drive. A RAW image file requires about 10 times more disc space than a high-quality JPEG! For example, a 16 GB SD card can store around 4,500 high quality JPEG images but only 450 in RAW format. Some high-end cameras have two memory card slots with various options, one being the ability to take and store JPEG images on one and RAW files on the other.

On the flash system

- Use the Mode button to select E-TTL for Canon, TTL, or TTL-BL for Nikon to allow fully automatic flash illumination (See the information window on the flash)
- Confirm the flash output of each tube is 1:1

Most dental photography is 'close-up' where the depth of field is paramount. This is maximised by using the smallest practical aperture, (large number) and f22 is suggested.

Many systems will allow an aperture choice even smaller than f22, whilst in theory using these smaller apertures would increase the depth of field, it is understood that using extremely small apertures in current DSLR (digital single-lens reflex), diffraction can occur with a resultant degradation of the image. For this reason, the author suggests a minimum aperture of f22.

Using the camera

Metering area

Automatic exposure systems base their calculations from various areas of the subject and centre-weighted average or spot metering is the suggested preset. The choice is available under 'Metering Mode' in the shooting set-up menu. **Figure 7** shows the following options on a Canon 200D: Evaluative, Partial, Spot, and Centre-weighted average, with Spot metering selected. Please note these options can vary from model-to-model and make-to-make.

Intra- and peri-oral views

Assuming the cameras are set as above, the only variable settings are the choice of aperture and field of view.

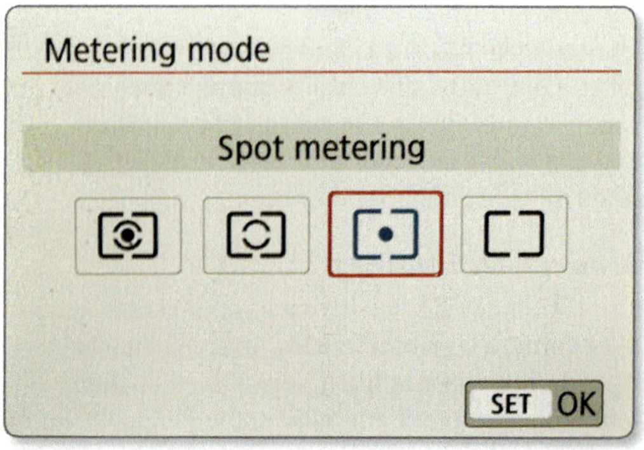

Figure 7 Metering modes.

Aperture

- Select f22

Field of view

For consistency of image size, it is suggested that the field of view is preselected by setting the magnification ratio in/on the lens barrel and achieving focus whilst holding the camera at eye level and moving the whole assembly until focus is achieved. As the distance between lens and subject is quite short, it is well worth practicing with a plaster model or similar initially.

Magnification ratios

These are the numbers, usually in yellow as shown in **Figure 8**, which set the magnification ratios for close-up photography. These macro lenses were designed and calibrated for 35 mm cameras and the ratios shown refer to the ratio between the subject size in life to the image size on the film, now sensor. Thus at 1:1 the image on the film or full frame sensor would be the same size as the subject (**Figure 9**) and at 1:2 as shown in **Figure 10** the image would be 1/2 life size. They refer to the ratio of the subject size in life to the image size on the sensor. They are calibrated originally for 35 mm film and now for full frame sensor cameras. A full frame sensor measures 24 × 36 mm compared with the cropped sensor APS-C (Advanced Photo System type-C) sizes of 23.7 × 15.5 mm (Nikon) and 25.1 × 16.7 mm (Canon). In practice, the difference between fields of view with Nikon or Canon cropped sensor cameras can be considered insignificant.

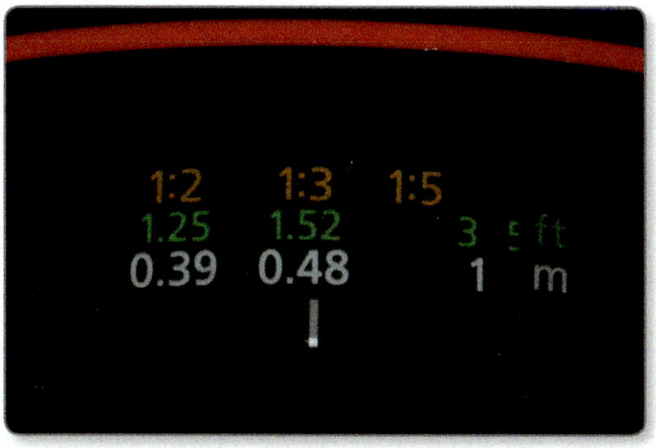

Figure 8 Magnification ratios in yellow.

As most readers will be using cameras with smaller APS-C sensors these numbers should be used as a reference rather than a true mathematical ratio (**Figure 8**) (Please note that this image was photographed using the 'polar_eyes' filter to eliminate the glare from the lens' 'window.').

Crop factor

Figures 9 and **10** show the field of view with 100 mm macro lens set at 1:1 and 1:2 on a full frame sensor camera. At this setting, the images on the sensor are true-life and half-life size images of the subject.

However, the sensors in the popular DSLR cameras are smaller than their full frame counterparts and thus the settings on the lens do not correlate with the images when comparing formats and setting 1:1 and 1:2 on a cropped sensor camera would give the images as shown in **Figure 11** in the black frames.

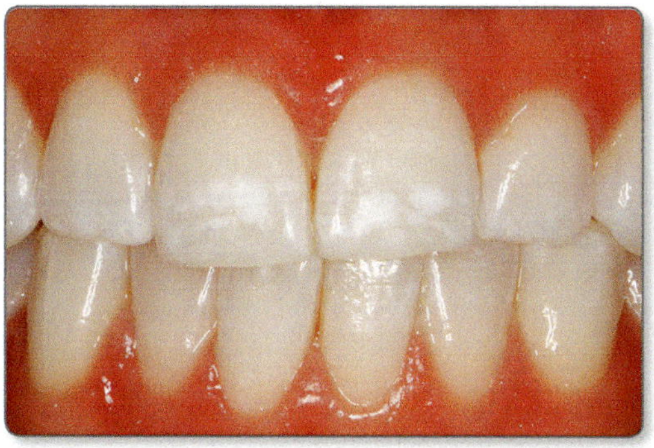

Figure 9 Magnification ratio set @ 1:1 on full frame camera.

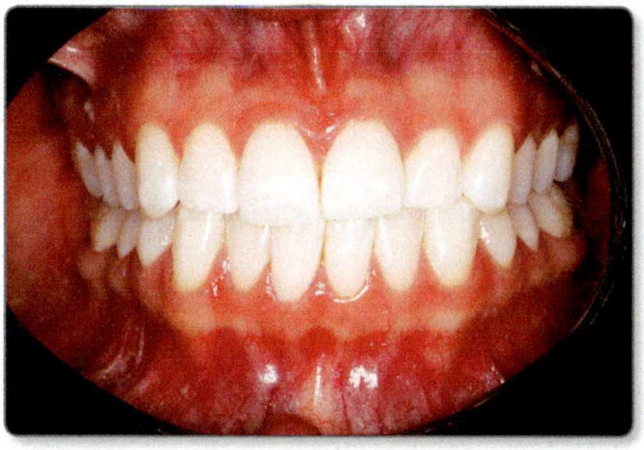

Figure 10 Magnification ratio set @ 1:2 on full frame camera.

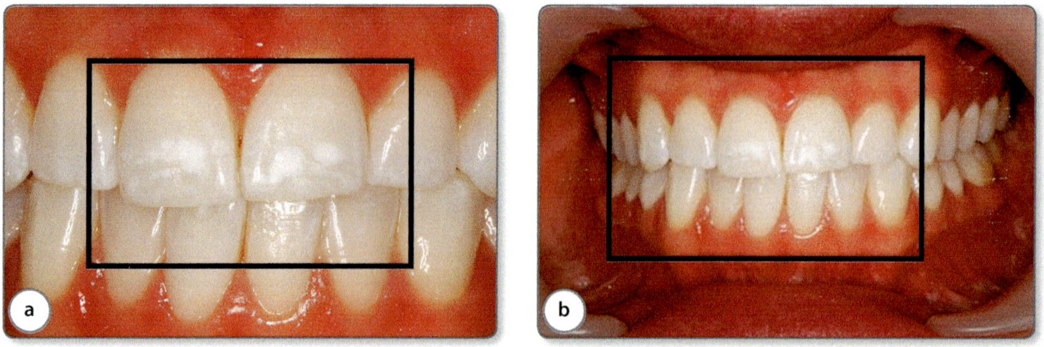

Figure 11 (a) Image achieved with cropped sensor camera with magnification ratio set at 1:1 and (b) with ratio set at 1:2.

Restorative and orthodontic dentistry

These procedures probably account for most images taken and have been singled out as there is a specific requirement for successive images to be the same size and in the same place.

Consistency in fields of view

The only way to achieve consistent images sizes with DSLR photography is to maintain the same camera to subject distance. This means presetting the field of view on the lens and moving the camera assembly whilst looking through the viewfinder until the subject is in focus. Using DSLRs with APS-C sensors the following guidelines are considered acceptable. Most cameras also offer a 'grid' screen which facilitates orientation.

Presetting the lens ratio on cropped sensor cameras (see Figure 12)

Generally,

- 1:1—will give a two upper central view
- 1:1.5—will give a four upper anterior view
- 1:2.5—will give an upper six anterior view
- 1:3—will give a commissure-to-commissure or full arch view (**Figure 12**)

Facial photography

The easiest way to standardise facial views is to have a fixed position for the patient. The photographer should be approximately

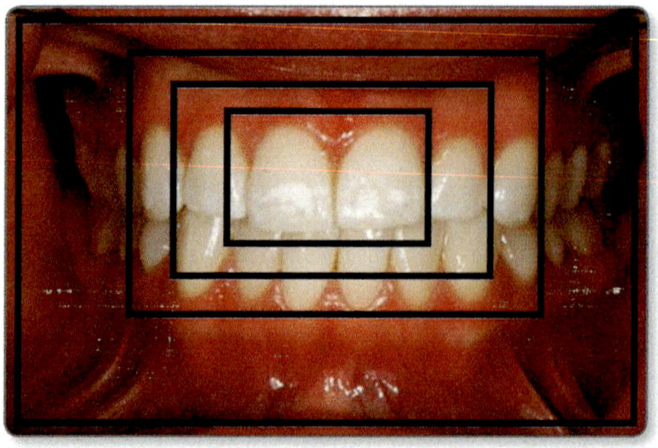

Figure 12 Settings on copped sensor camera. 1:1 two centrals, 1:1.5 four upper anteriors, 1:2.5 canine-to-canine, 1:3 full arch.

2 metres (6 ½ feet) away and using manual focus (MF), find the exact distance where the patient's head fills the frame. Once this point is noted all facial views will be near enough the same size. If autofocus is selected, the face will be focused from a variety of distances and image sizes will vary. It is of course possible to use autofocus if the operator and subject are always the same distance apart. However, the operator must remember to revert to MF for consistency in the clinical shots.

Autofocus

There are situations where image capture is more important than consistency of field of view with oral surgery and implantology being prime examples. In these circumstances autofocus might be the preferred setting.

Until this point, eye level photography has been emphasised but in the above situations both camera and operator can intrude into the operating field. One option to alleviate this aspect is to select live view (LV) on the camera and use

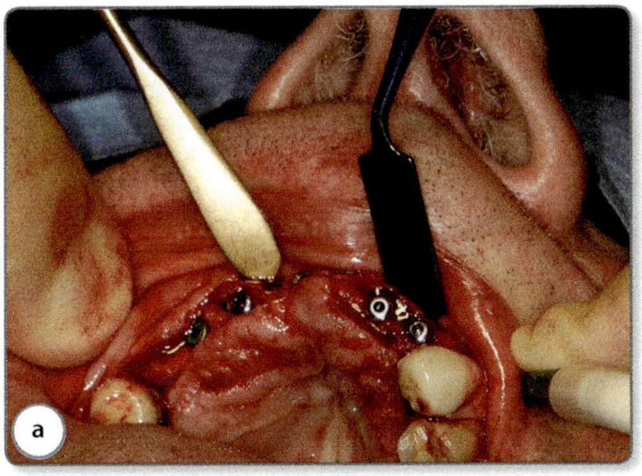
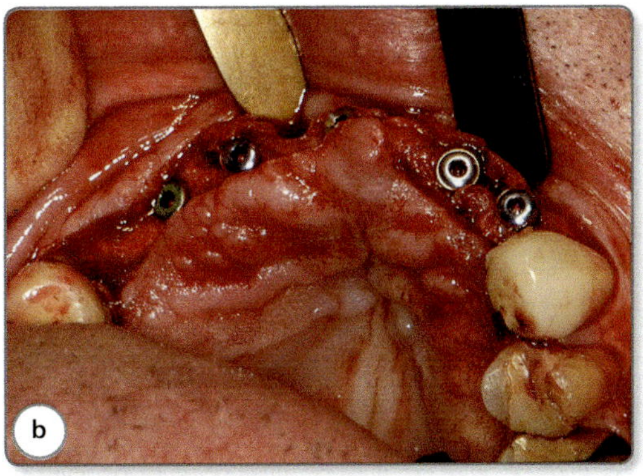

Figures 13a and b Original image and cropped image. (*Courtesy:* Dr E Scher) (*Photography:* Dr Peter Gordon)

the rear screen as the viewfinder. If the system is not too bulky, one-handed operation may be possible; in which case the operator should have a wrist strap as a safety precaution.

Figure 13 was taken holding the camera with one hand and using the rear screen as the viewfinder. Autofocus was selected and there was minimal intrusion for the surgeon. Admittedly there was extraneous material in the original shot but cropping this out was easy.

Consent

Before any photographic image is taken, signed consent must be obtained from the patient or legal guardian, etc. Images form part of the patient's clinical records and as such appropriate security and confidentiality must be observed. The following template has been taken from the web and can be considered suitable.

CONSENT TO DENTAL PHOTOGRAPHY

I, ______________________________ (Patient), authorise Dr. ______________________________ (Dentist), to take photographs, and/or videos of my face, jaws and teeth, before, during and after treatment.

I consent to allow the photographs to be used for the following (*delete any that are not applicable)

**Dental records, dental research, dental education including lectures, seminars, demonstrations, professional publications such as journals or books*

**Marketing material, including websites and printed materials, patient education *FULL FACE/*MOUTH*

I further understand that if the photographs and/or videos are used, my name or other identifying information will be kept confidential, (other than if Full Face photographs are used)

I do not expect compensation, financial or otherwise, for the use of these photographs.

Signature (Dentist) ______________________________

Signature (Patient) ______________________________Date ____________

www.photographyfordentists.com/resources/dental-photography-consent-form.doc

5 Other systems

Introduction

It is generally accepted that the bench-mark standard for clinical photography is based on the Single Lens Reflex body. The main criticisms are invariably based on complexity and bulk. Hopefully, the preceding chapters have eliminated the concerns on the former. As far as weight is concerned, the lens always will be the major factor, but lighter bodies and flash systems are covered in Chapter 6.

There is always a small demand for cameras that are smaller, lighter and "less complicated." This chapter will cover some current alternatives.

Mirrorless cameras

Professional photographers are increasingly turning to mirrorless cameras both in the full frame and cropped sensor bodies. When comparing like for like on specifications, the mirrorless bodies currently tend to be considerably more expensive than 'DSLR' (digital single-lens reflex). There are a few bodies at entry level prices and no doubt this will increase in due course. As far as the author is concerned the camera must have an eye level viewfinder and this restricts the choice even further. The Canon EOS M50 is an entry level, cropped sensor, mirrorless body with an eye level viewfinder that works automatically when the camera is raised to the eye. The lens mount is specific to this type of body and the range of lenses is limited. However, an adaptor EF-EOS M, will enable a full range of Canon lenses to be used. Whilst the M50 is slightly smaller than the DSLR 250D (**Figures 1** and **2**) it is only 2.3 oz (60 g) lighter and this is totally offset when the 100 mm macro, lens mount adaptor and flash system is added. The inbuilt flash will not trigger the Metz MS-1 so that another trigger will need to be used, e.g. the Canon EL 100 flash. In conclusion, if one is looking for a lightweight system, the cropped sensor mirrorless route is not the answer. At the time of writing, no other mirrorless body in the genre will trigger the Metz MS-1 flash with the camera's built in flash. In the author's opinion, eye level photography is a must for the majority of close-up dental photography and whilst the M50's eye level viewfinder is excellent and instantaneous in switching from the screen view, the image is harder to focus than with the direct view from a DSLR and unlike a DSLR the 'just taken' image remains in the viewfinder instead of the original subject. In addition, the cost of the adaptor for the 100 mm macro lens is almost half the cost of the lens.

Four thirds system

The 'Four Thirds System' is a standard created by Olympus and Eastman Kodak for DSLR camera

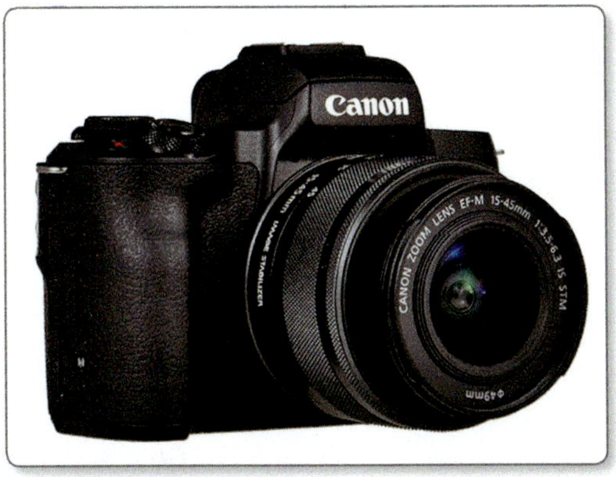

Figure 1 Canon M50 mirrorless.

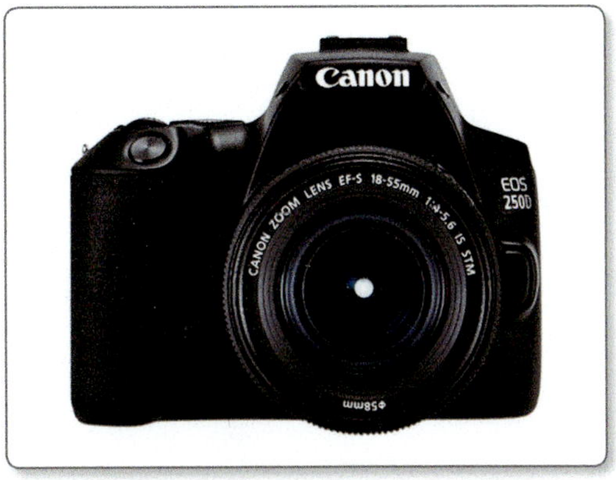

Figure 2 Canon 250D DSLR.

and mirrorless camera design and development. The sensor size for these cameras is 17.3 × 13 mm compared with 22.2 × 14.8 mm for the Canon-cropped sensor cameras.

The smaller sensor has enabled the system to be much smaller and lighter than DSLRs. At the time of writing only Olympus produce a suitable macro lens and flash system. However, all manufacturers following this system incorporate a standard lens mount thus allowing interchangeability of lenses. The crop factor is 1:2, and therefore, setting the magnification ratio on the lens at 1:4 a full arch image can be captured. **Figure 3** shows the comparison in size between a DSLR set-up and the Olympus.

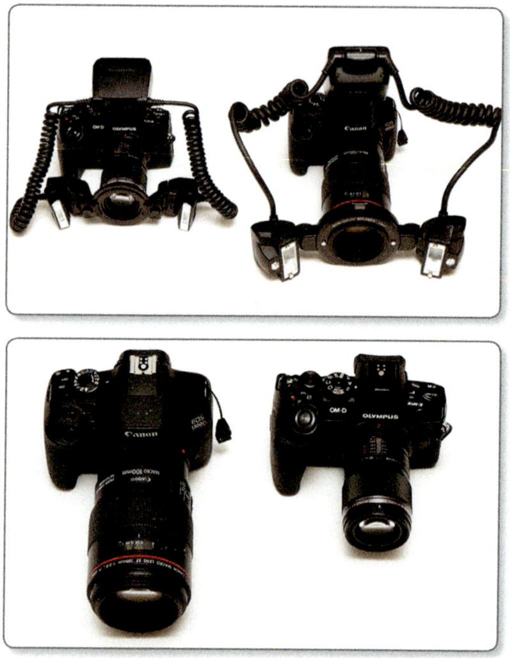

Figure 3 Comparative sizes of Olympus and Canon systems.

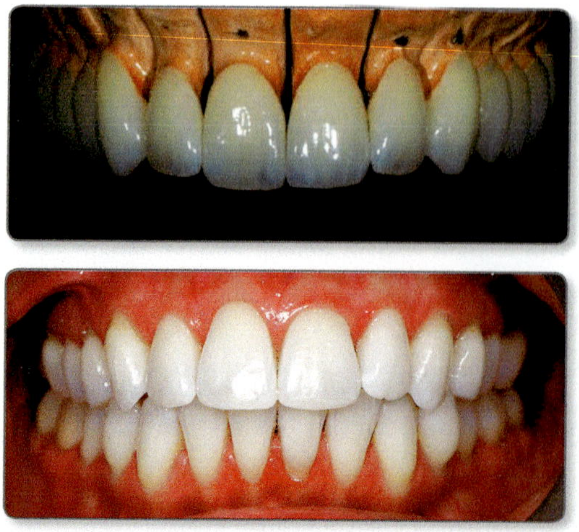

Figure 4 Images taken with Olympus system.

If you are looking for the smallest lightest system closest to a DSLR, the Olympus set-up might be worth considering. Working with eye level electronic viewfinders takes a little getting used to especially as with the Canon M50 it shows the 'just taken' image as opposed to the original subject (**Figure 4**). Also, the lens defaults to the infinity setting when the camera is turned 'OFF' and the magnification ratio therefore, needs resetting every time prior to use. Whilst the 60 mm macro lens and twin flash are similar in price to the DSLR units, the Olympus bodies currently tend to be more expensive but no doubt prices will drop as they become more popular.

Cameras specifically designed for dental use

This is a brief introduction as to what is available and not a full 'road test.'

Shofu CIII

At the time of writing, (March, 2020) the CIII was to be replaced by the CIIII. It is understood that the major differences are that it has image stabilisation and 4k movie facility. The basic design remains unchanged.

The Shofu CIII has been designed specifically for dental photography which it performs excellently (**Figure 5**). It is a compact lightweight unit easily held one-handed with the rear screen

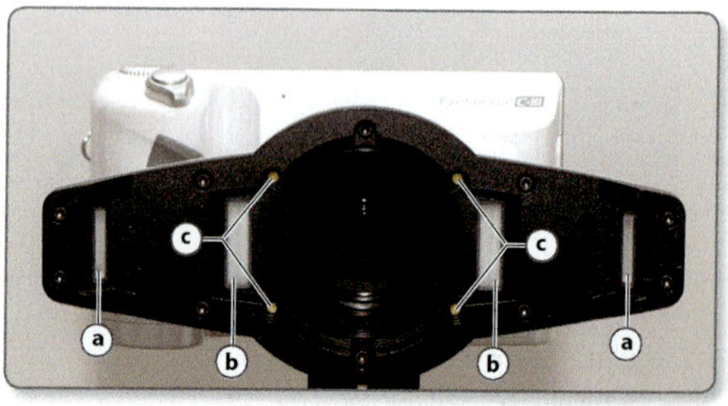

Figure 5 (a) Outer flash; (b) Inner flash; (c) One of four focussing LEDs.

acting as the viewfinder. It is capable of repetitive same size images using the pre-sets in the camera menu (**Figures 6** to **9**). These pre-sets accessed via the rear touchscreen are:

- Standard
- Surgery
- Mirror
- Face
- Low glare
- Whitening
- Tele-Macro
- Isolate shade

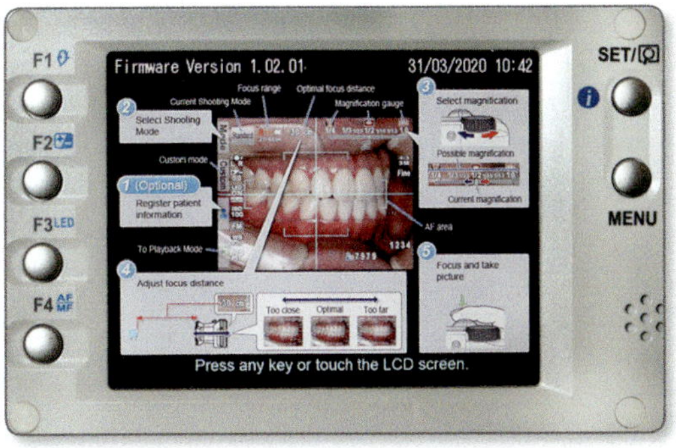

Figure 6 Start-up screen.

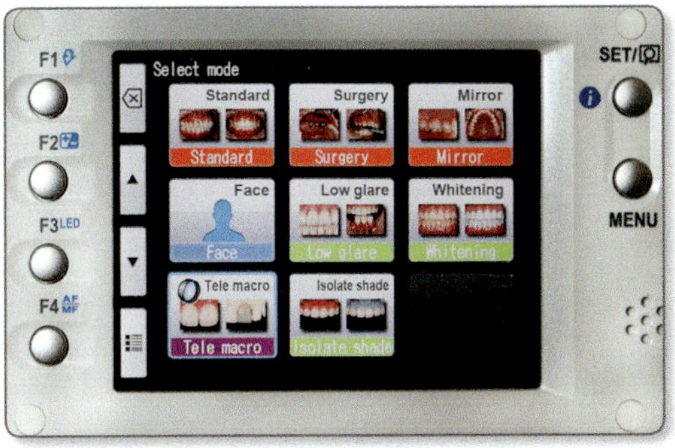

Figure 7 Menu selection screen showing eight pre-sets.

Standard views

Standard is the choice for routine photography with a selection range from part face to four teeth, as in **Figure 8**. The choices are labelled as: 1/4, 1/3, 1/1.25, 1/2, 1/1,5, 1/1.3, and 1/1. These fields of view correspond with ratios used for full frame cameras and do not represent the ratios of subject to image sizes on this sensor. Thus 1:1 will correspond to four upper anterior teeth and 1:2 a full arch. Having selected the field of view(see **Figure 8**), the operator has two focusing choices. He/she can move the camera using the rear screen to focus until the image is sharp, and then take the picture. This distance will be fixed according to the ratio chosen. The alternative method is to use the 'AUTO-CROP' facility, position the camera within the range shown on the screen and use the 'AUTOFOCUS.' This function produces same size images from a small range of camera positions. The four LEDs illuminate the subject when the shutter button is depressed, but the subject is illuminated by either the inner or outer flash tubes depending on the setting.

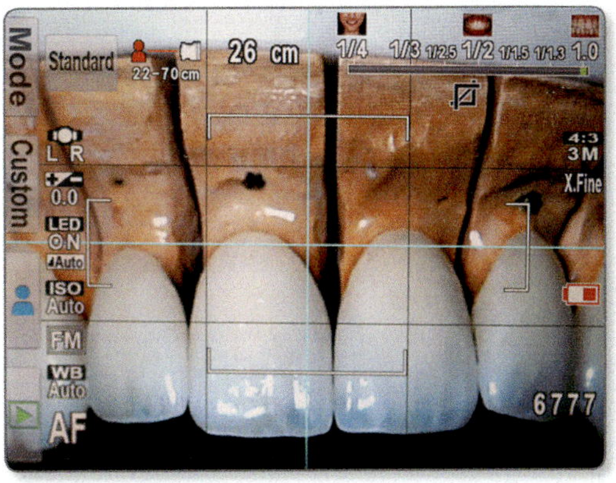

Figure 8 Ratio choice in standard setting.

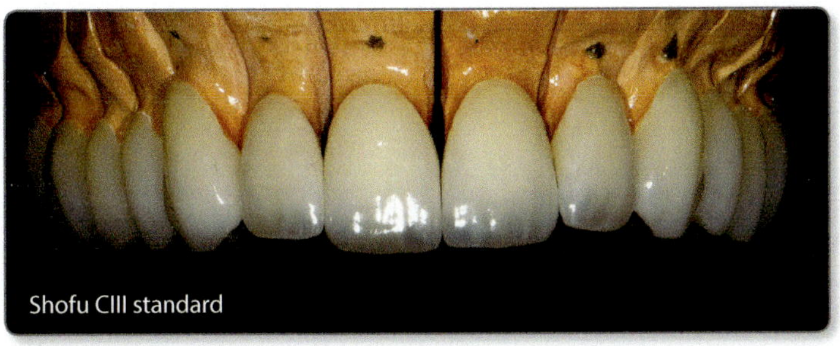

Figure 9 Image achieved with setting at ½ see Figure 8.

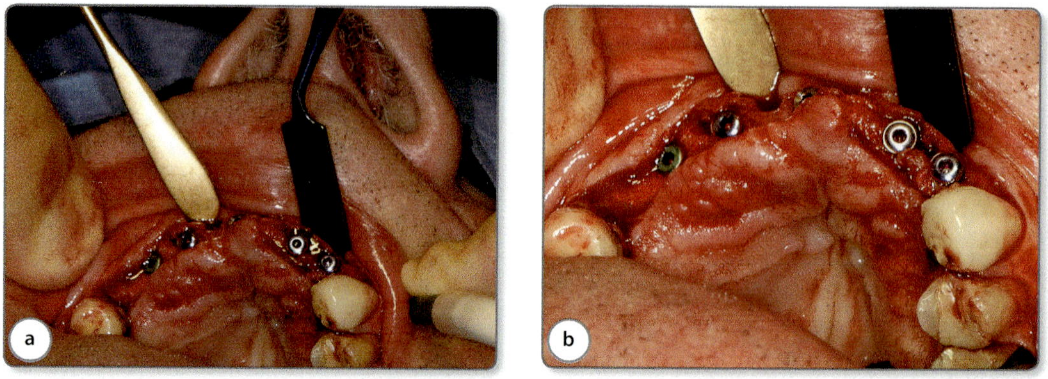

Figures 10a and b Original image.
(*Courtesy:* Surgeon Dr E Scher, Photograph Dr P Gordon)

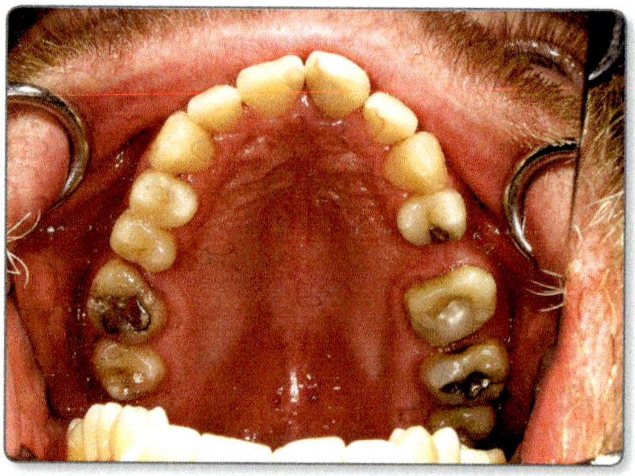

Figure 11 Upper arch taken with Shofu camera.

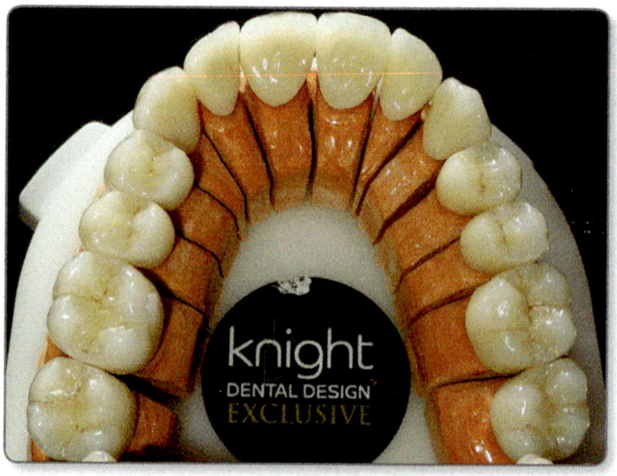

Figure 12 Mirror image has been flipped horizontally.

Surgery setting

The surgery setting allows the previous selection of images to be attained from approximately twice the distance. This mode is extremely useful in the surgical field where one can hold just the camera over the operation field, select the field of view on the rear screen, and use auto focus. The images may not be constant in size but can be easily cropped subsequently (see **Figures 10a** and **b**).

These images are illuminated by the outside flash tubes.

Mirror

This view automatically flips the image and converts the laterally inverted picture to be anatomically correct (**Figure 12**).

Face

The manufacturer suggests these images are taken with the camera in the vertical position. Auto cropping is not available in this setting (**Figures 13** and **14**).

Low glare and whitening

Figures 15 to **17** are illuminated by the less intense inner flashes and reduce the intensity of the high light glare.

The standard view is included for comparison.

Tele-Macro

Close-ups of individual teeth can be taken using a supplementary lens screwed in front of the standard lens (**Figure 18**).

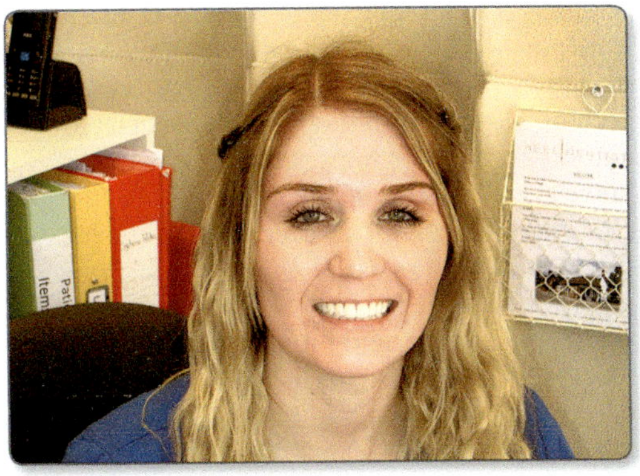

Figure 13 Facial view in surgery.

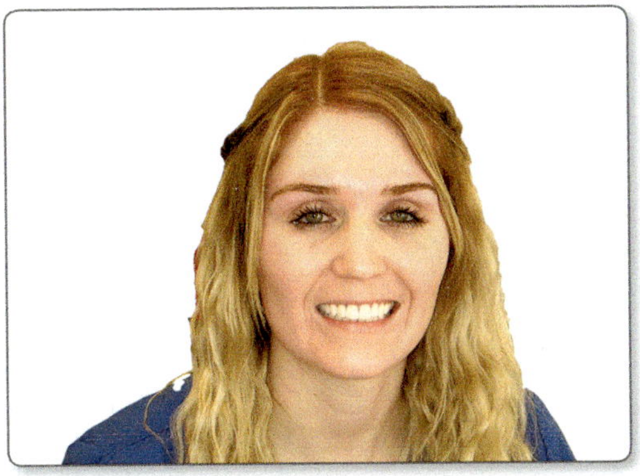

Figure 14 Background 13 removed using "PHOTOSCISSORS" software.

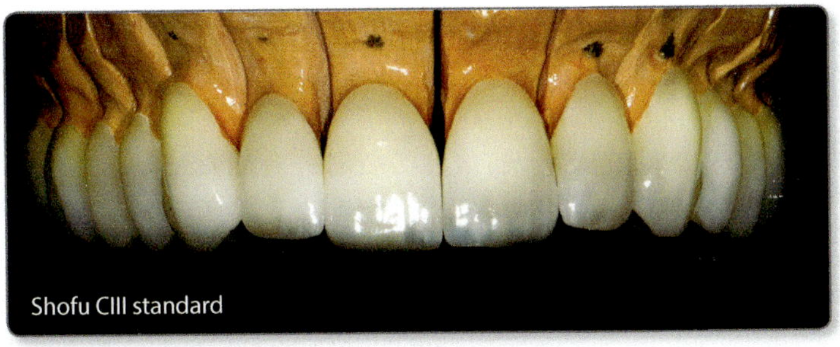

Figure 15 Standard illumination.

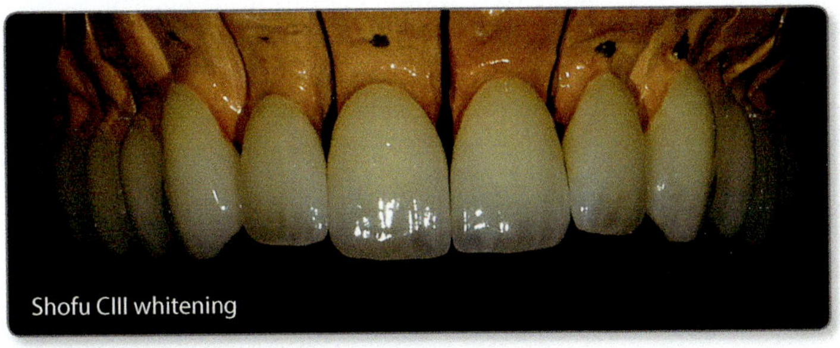

Figure 16 Whitening illumination.

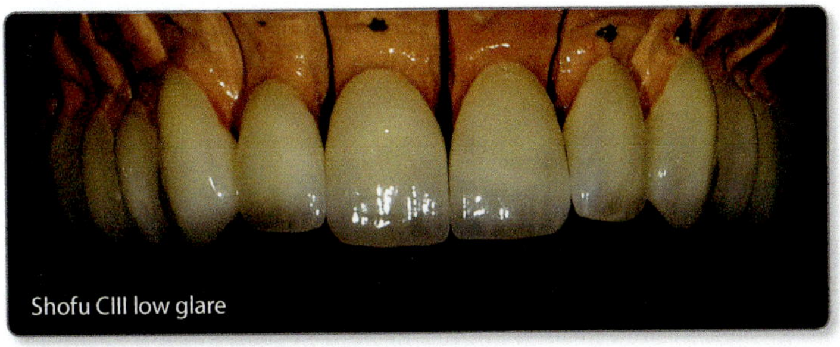

Figure 17 Low glare illumination.

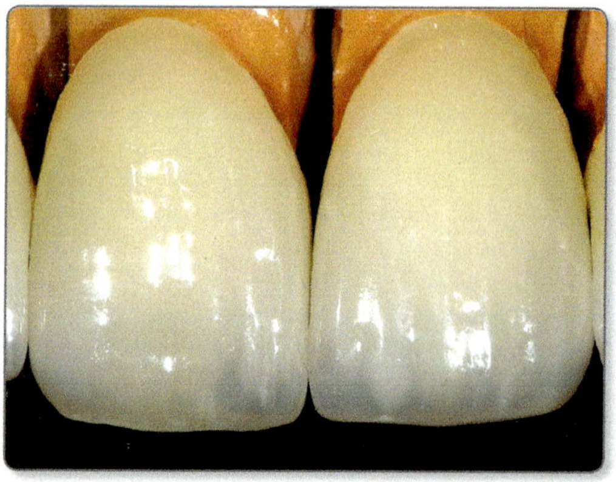

Figure 18 Image using Tele-Macro lens.

Isolate shade

This is a novel function allowing the production of a normal image and one where the teeth are reproduced in their natural colour and the surrounding tissues in monochrome (**Figures 19** and **20**).

The images are captured and stored on SD cards. If these are formatted by the camera, they will be compatible with the Shofu management software which is a free download.

There is no doubt that this lightweight unit fulfils the task beautifully. The potential user will have to decide if all the available facilities to justify the price tag.

Dentaleyepad

This novel unit is based on a Samsung phone and in common with the Shofu camera the rear screen acts as the viewfinder (**Figure 21**). There is no memory card, the images are immediately downloaded to a computer. The camera can be set to retain the images, up to 2000, or deleted automatically following a successful transfer. There is an indicator on the screen which confirms a successful transfer. If unsuccessful, the image will be retained. In order to facilitate repetitive images, the camera is pre-loaded with overlays/templates and the user simply lines up the patient's teeth with the outlines. There are pre-set overlays in set sequences for different requirements such as the AACD (American Academy of Cosmetic Dentistry)/BACD (British Academy of Cosmetic Dentistry, orthodontists, etc. Or the user can set-up their own series (**Figure 22**).

As with the Shofu, this camera is packed with additional functions.

Dinecorp

Dinecorp in the US have modified compact cameras for dental use for many years. Currently, this is the Olympus 'Toughie' which is totally waterproof and therefore, easily disinfected (**Figure 23**).

Like the Shofu and Dentaleyepad, and in common with most compact cameras, the rear screen is used to focus the subject. It is very simple to use but it is not easy to achieve same size repetitive images using the autofocus system. Whilst capable of capturing excellent images, there will always be slightly uneven lighting as the flash is to one side of the lens (**Figures 24** to **28**).

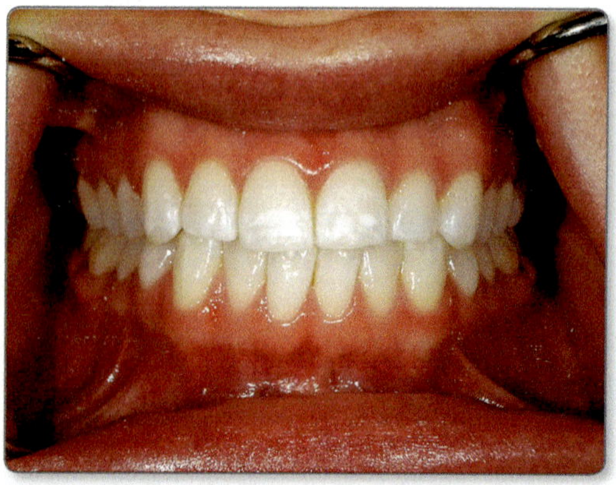

Figure 19 Standard view

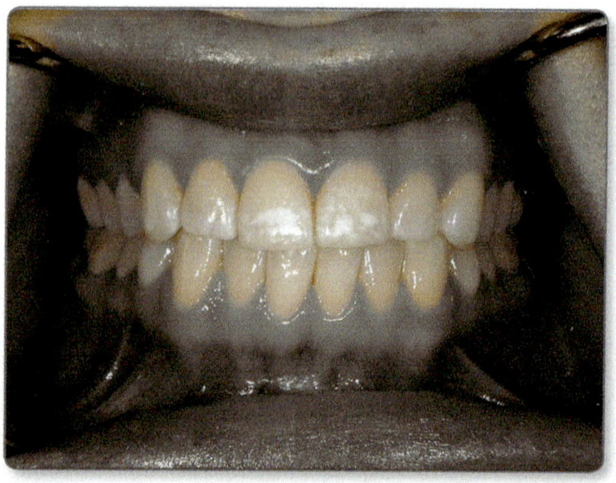

Figure 20 Isolate shade image.

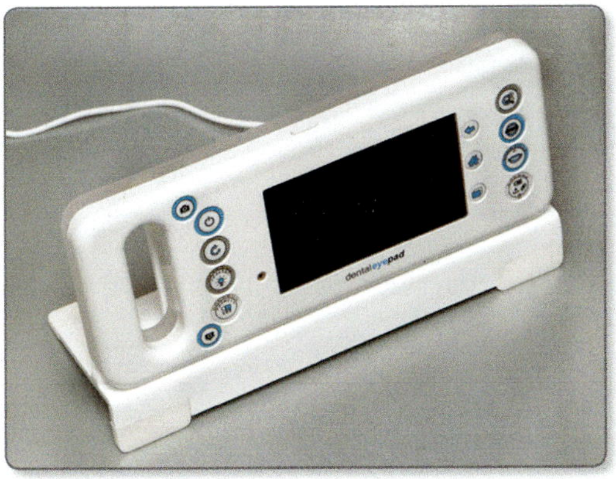

Figure 21 Dentaleyepad on charging stand.

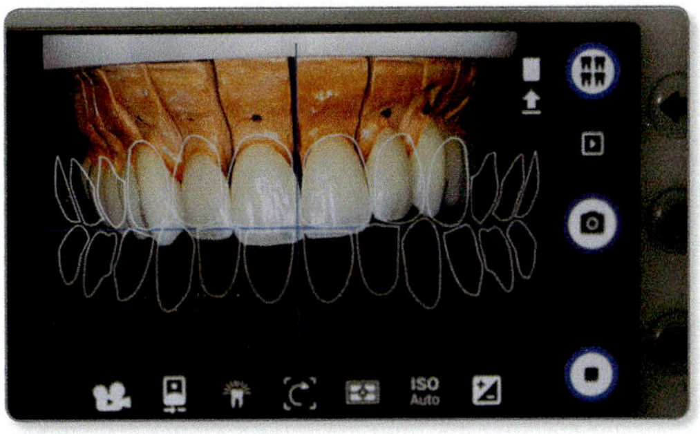

Figure 22 Screen showing overlay for anterior image.

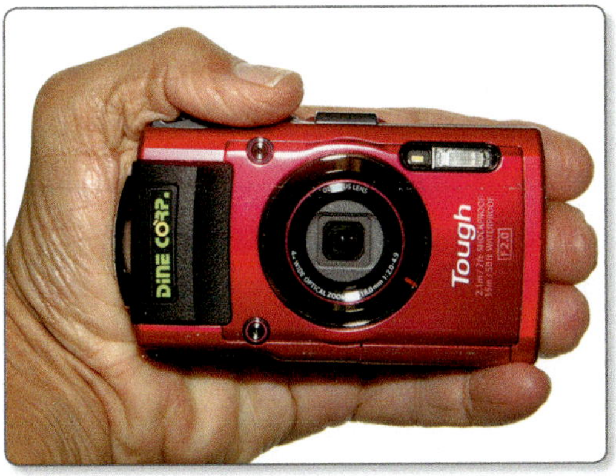

Figure 23 Dine camera.
(*Courtesy:* Dine Corps)

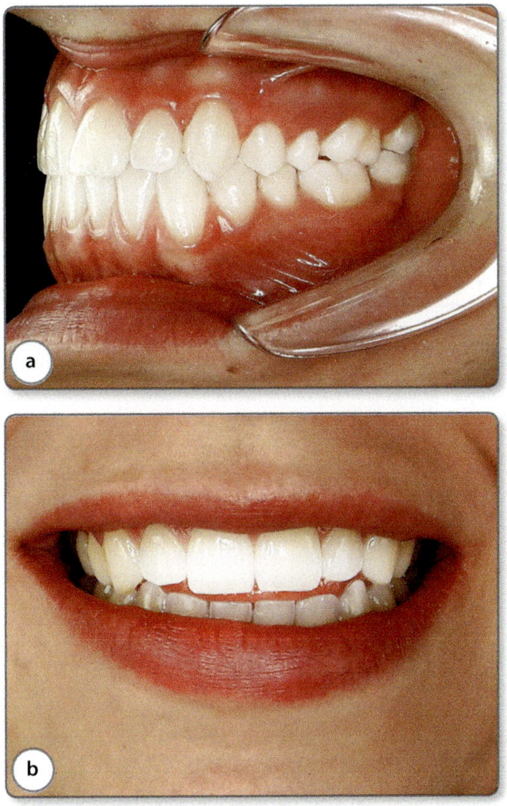

Figures 24a and b Clinical images using dine camera.
(*Courtesy:* Dine Corps)

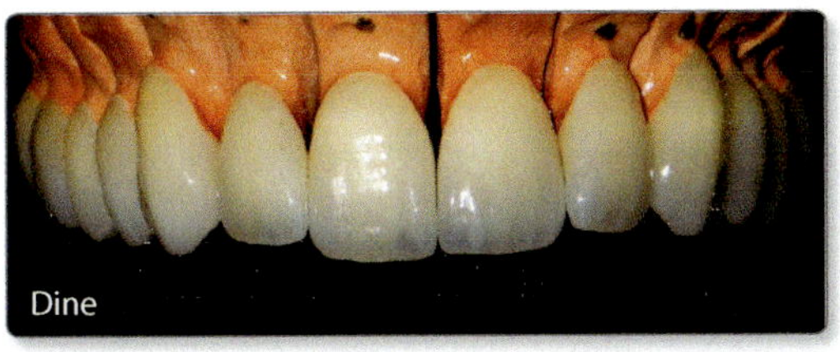

Figure 25 Image of static model showing uneven lighting due to off centre flash taken by the Dr P Gordon.

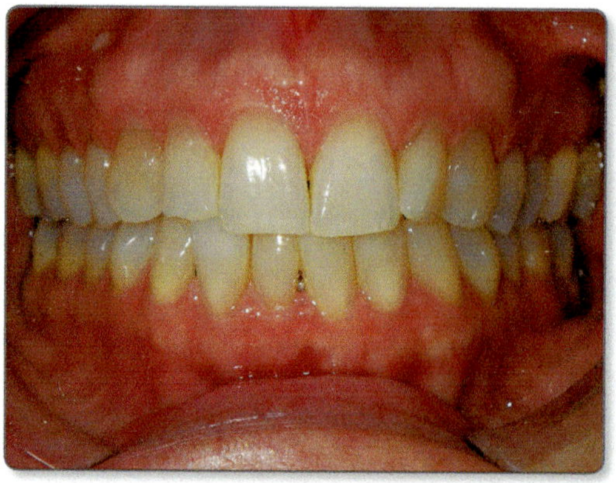

Figure 26 Clinical Image using dine camera. (*Courtesy:* Dine Corps)

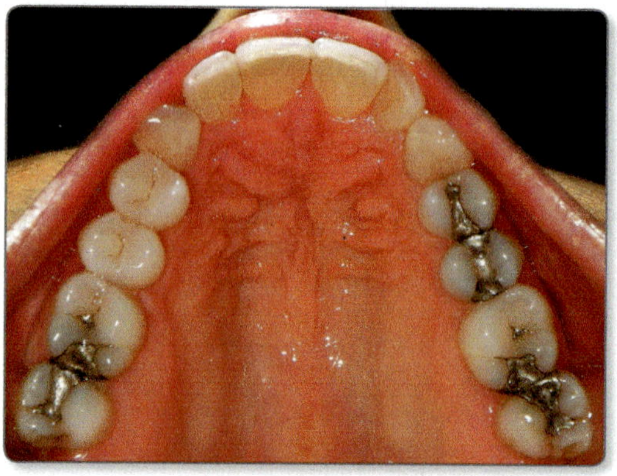

Figure 27 Clinical image using dine camera. (*Courtesy:* Dine Corps)

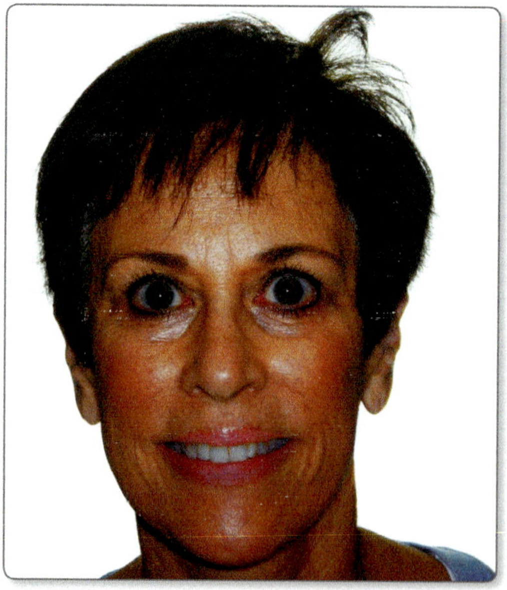

Figure 28 Clinical image using dine camera. (*Courtesy:* Dine Corps)

They also produce a ring light and pistol grip for mobile phones and a small ring light for eyepads (**Figure 29**).

Mobile dental photography

The mobile dental photography (MDP) system was designed by Professor Louis Hardan DDS, CES, DEA, PhD and is now produced by Smile Line. It is basically a very versatile lighting system that can be securely attached to any smart phone between 55 mm and 85 mm in width. The LED lighting system can produce similar results to ring flash, twin flash, and soft box illumination. In addition, it includes accessories for cross polarising (**Figures 30** to **32**).

Mobile phones and protocol

There is no doubt that mobile phone use for clinical photography has increased exponentially over the last few years and certainly this will continue. What is probably most important to consider, is not the ability of the phone to record images, but the safety and security of those images. Which of course means complying with patient confidentiality and GDPR (General Data Protection Regulation) in the UK and whatever regulations are in place elsewhere.

To quote Ms Kristen Bottrell GDC July, 2019 (General Dental Council)

'We would consider *any image* taken of a patient during their care to form part of their clinical record.' Any image implies whether recognizable or not and will require permission for any use outside of the clinical records.

My research has suggested that all UK Hospital Trusts have mobile phone protocols, namely the availability of 'Trust' phones available to clinical staff. These are connected only to the hospital's IT system with images to be downloaded to the patient's records and immediately deleted from the phone. Some general dental practices have a similar procedure in place. Without doubt there are occasions when it is expedient to use personal mobiles. In these situations, it is

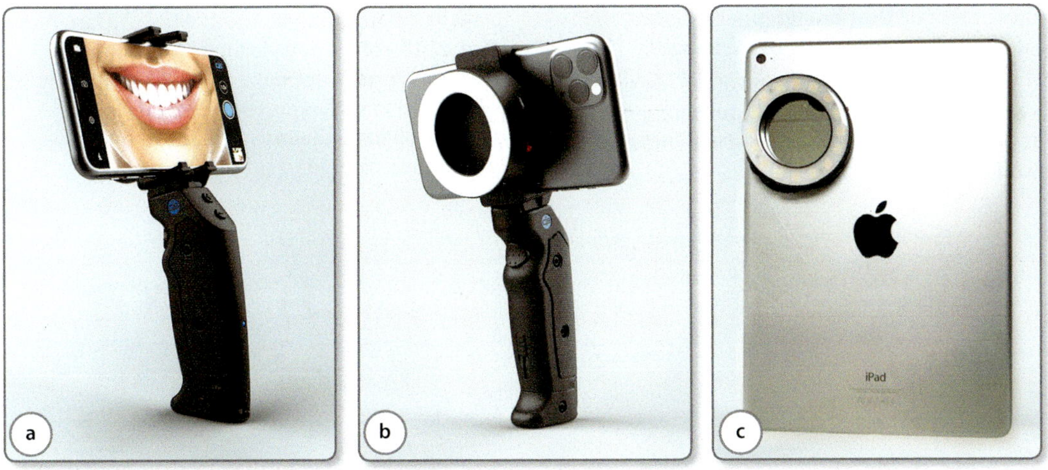

Figures 29a to c Pistol grip and ring light for mobile phones and iPad.

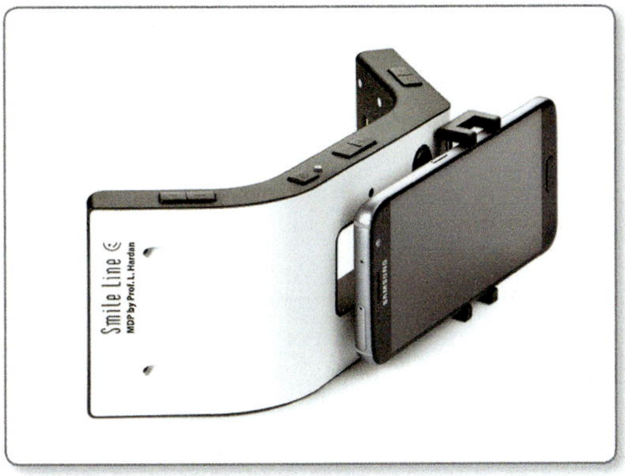

Figure 30 Mobile dental photography system.

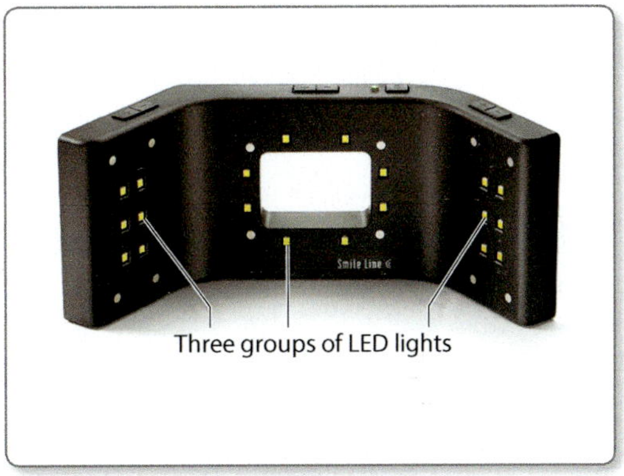

Figure 31 LED lighting system.

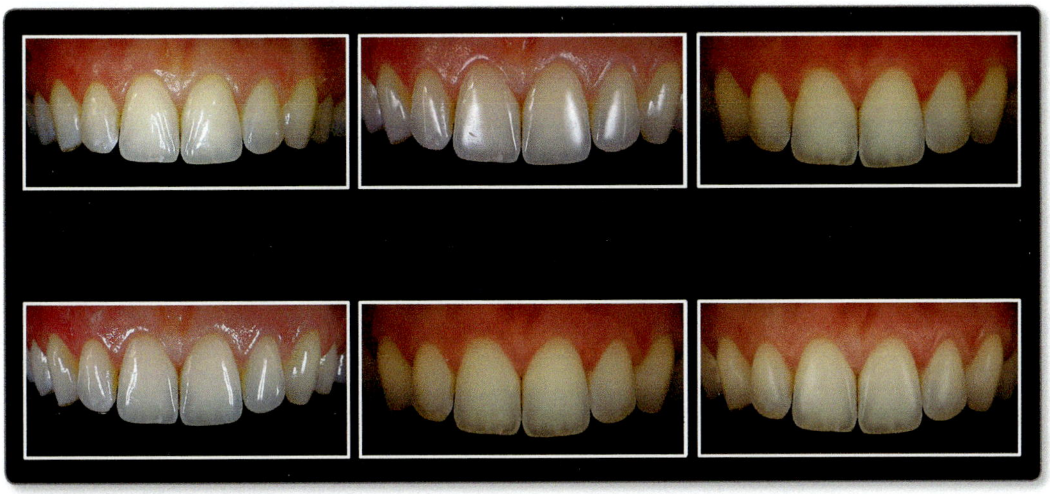

Figure 32 Images taken with MDP system.
(*Courtesy:* MDP system, Dr Louis Hardan and International Arab Journal of Dentistry, Volume 8 issue 3)

incumbent on the photographer to assure the safety and confidentiality of the images.

In the author's opinion one of the major shortcomings with mobile phone photography is that of perspective associated with the short working distances.

With reference to the Daily Mail of March 2nd, 2018, selfies have led to a 30% boom for rhinoplasty as noses appear to be unnaturally large both in selfies and other facial close-ups. **Figures 33** to **39** demonstrate the perspective problem as camera to subject distance lessens.

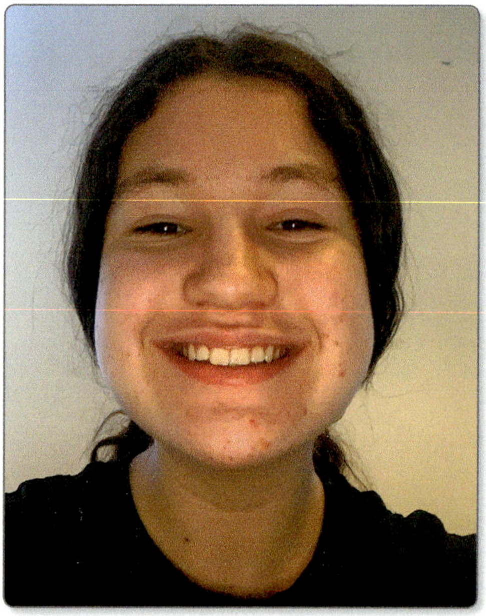

Figure 33 Mobile selfie.

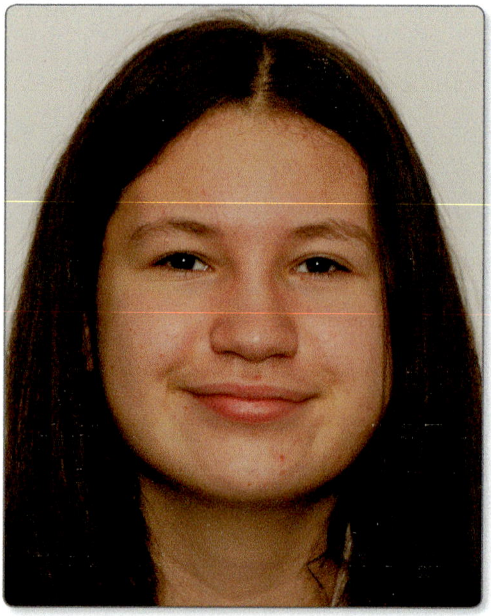

Figure 34 Image taken with standard DSLR set-up.

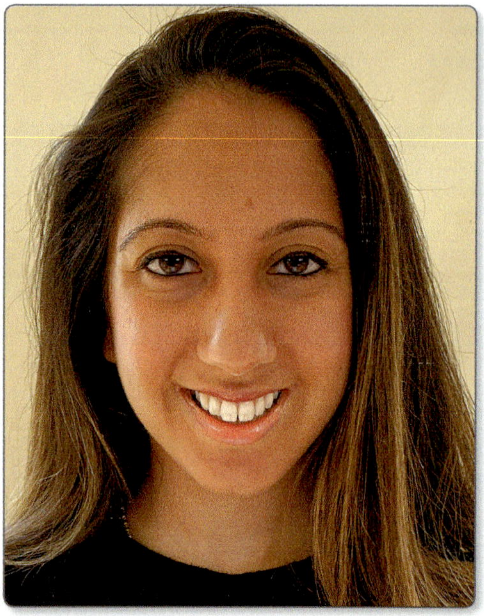

Figure 35 Mobile phone image.
(*Courtesy:* Dr Neel Jaiswal)

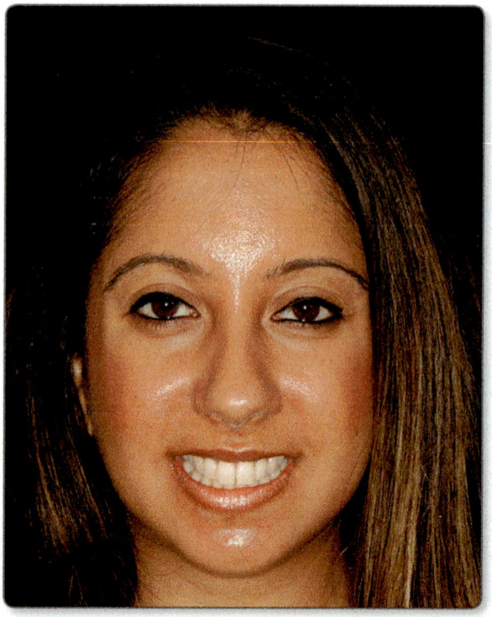

Figure 36 Image taken with standard DSLR set-up.
(*Courtesy:* Dr Neel Jaiswal)

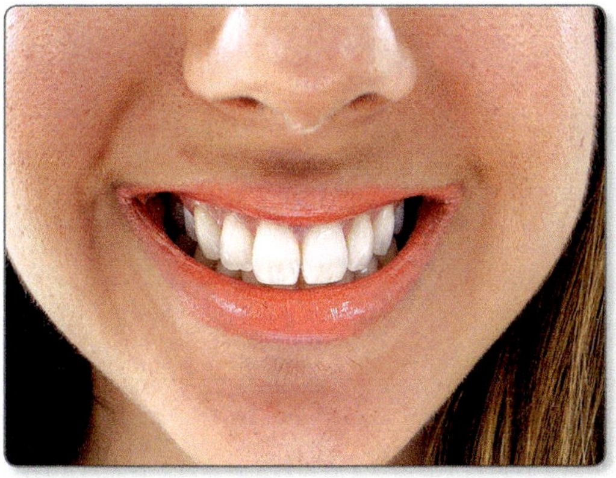

Figure 37 Phone image.
(*Courtesy:* Dr Neel Jaiswal)

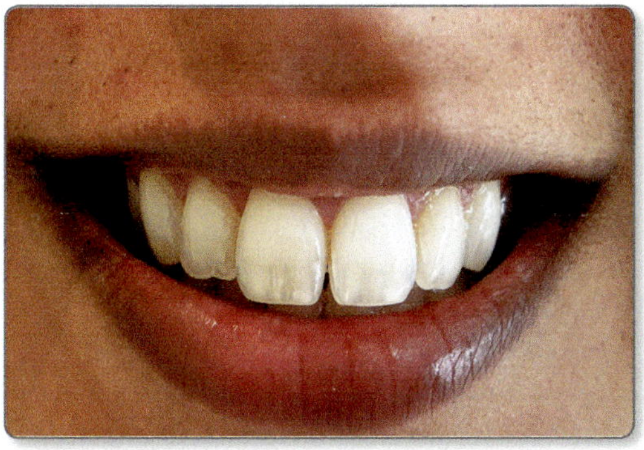

Figure 38 Mobile phone image.
(*Courtesy:* Dr Neel Jaiswal)

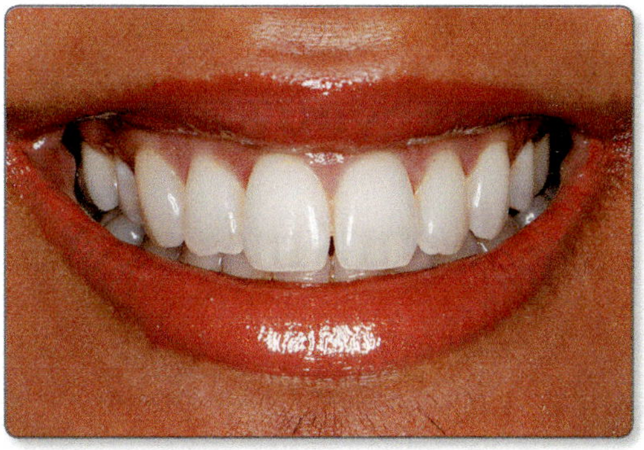

Figure 39 DSLR image.
(*Courtesy:* Dr Neel Jaiswal)

Photomicrography

This is really a totally different field, but a photographic record of an image taken via microscope can be just as important as any other image, and in this context a dedicated camera can be used. All microscopes have the ability to attach cameras and recommendations are probably best sought from the supplier. Generally, cameras with cropped sensors are the most common which gives a choice of DSLR or mirrorless. One of the biggest problems in this field is that of stabilisation as any movement of the patient no matter how slight can degrade the image and these systems do not have the ability to use electronic flash as illumination which can 'freeze' motion. In common with close-up photography the depth of field decreases with increases of magnification and at high magnification can be around 1 mm!

Figure 40 shows blood in a buccal canal indicating a perforation of the root.

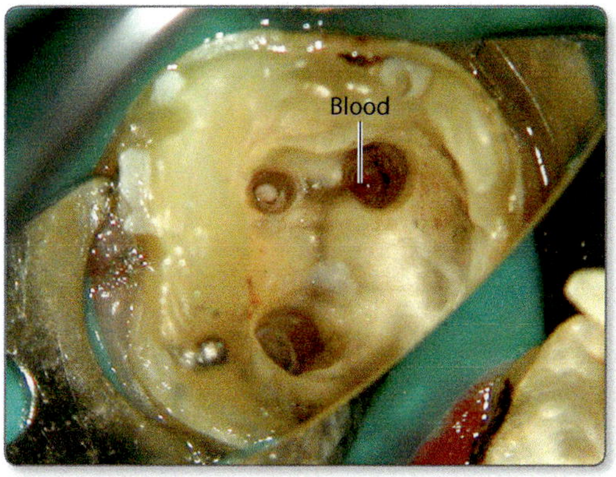

Figure 40 Blood in a buccal canal.
(*Courtesy:* Dr Tony Druttman)

6 Accessories

Introduction

The most important accessories are mirrors and retractors. The latter are available in plastic and metal and in a variety of sizes, colours, and designs - self-retaining, single-ended, and double-ended. While they are all autoclavable, plastic tends to discolour over time.

Direct photography

One simple piece of advice prior to dental photography, if applicable, is - 'to remove lipstick' (**Figure 1** and **2**).

The 'C'-shaped retractors are better for anterior views and 'V'-shaped for buccal views (**Figures 3** to **5**). When taking buccal views, always retract the opposite side to avoid the lip drooping in the middle.

Self-retaining retractors with tabs are very useful as they can be pushed/pulled to facilitate buccal views (**Figure 6**).

Retraction for occlusal views

Retractors and contrastors are readily available to facilitate occlusal views.

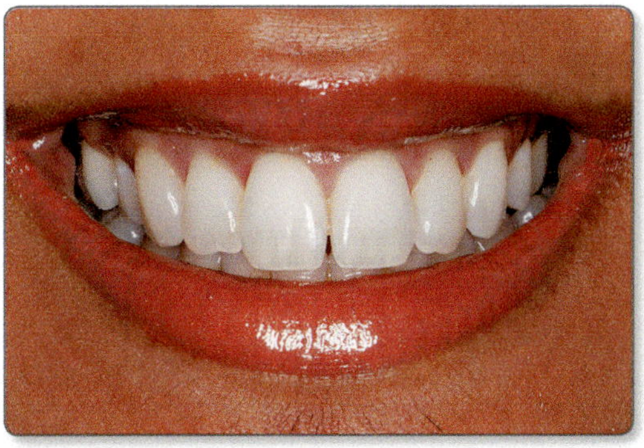

Figure 1 With lipstick.
(*Courtesy:* Dr Neel Jaiswal)

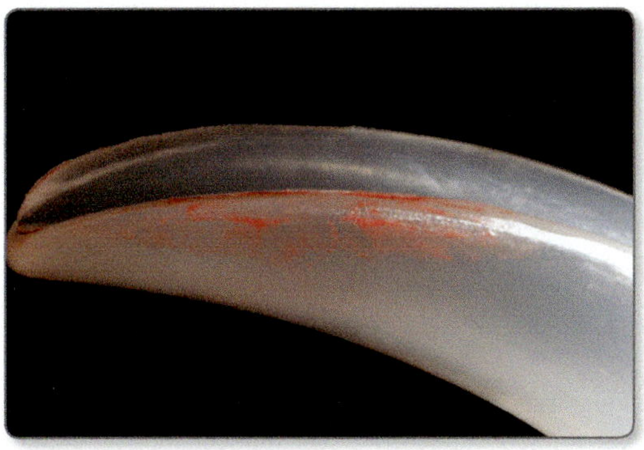

Figure 2 Lipstick on retractor.

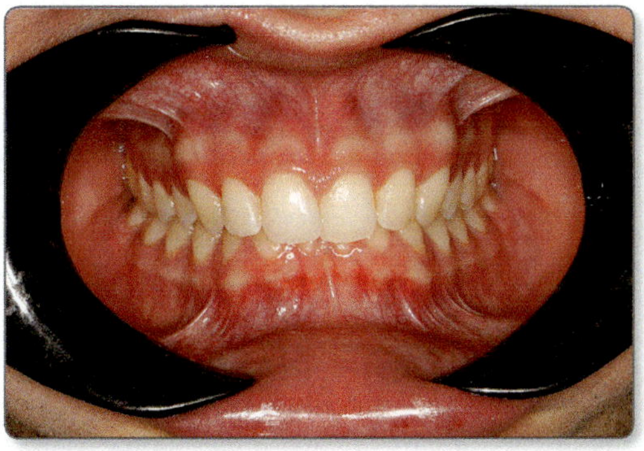

Figure 3 'C'-shaped retractors.
(*Courtesy:* Dr Neel Jaiswal)

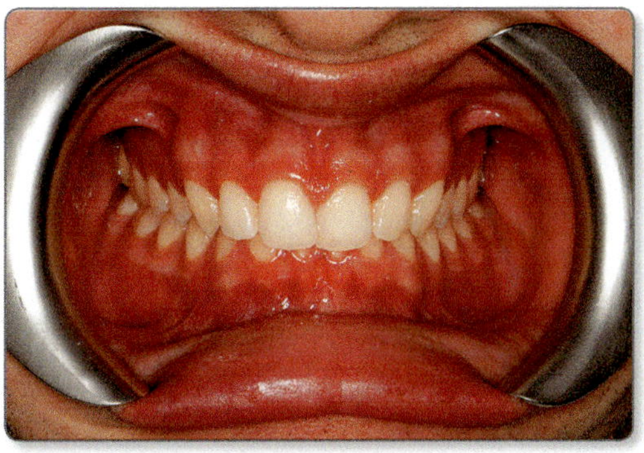

Figure 4 'Bracket'-shaped retractors.
(*Courtesy:* Dr Neel Jaiswal)

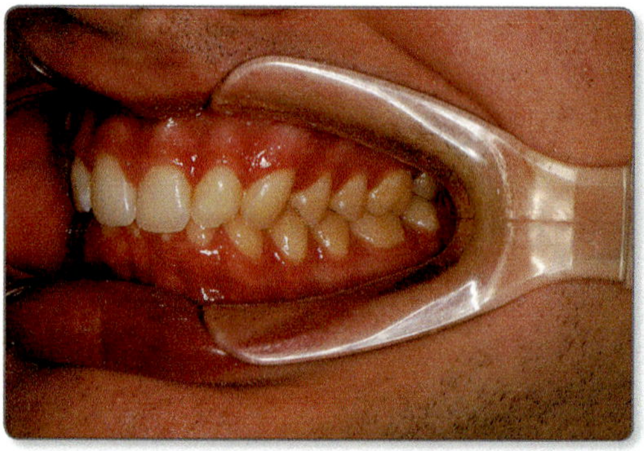

Figure 5 'V'-shaped retractor.
(*Courtesy:* Dr Neel Jaiswal)

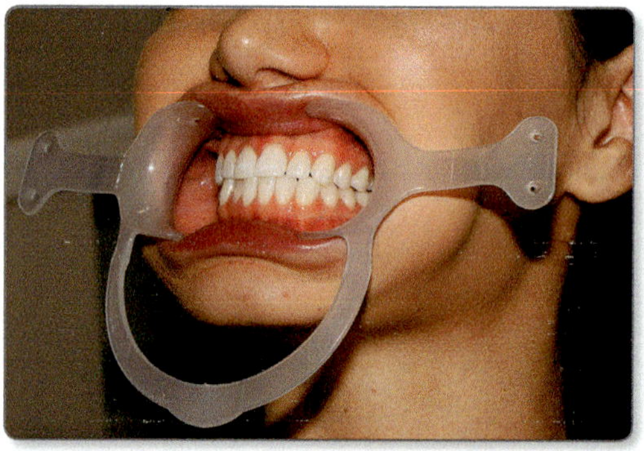

Figure 6 Self-retaining retractor with tabs.
(*Courtesy:* Dr Neel Jaiswal)

Oringer retractors

These self-retaining retractors come in three sizes and are very effective for anterior and occlusal views, as it is very easy to combine using these retractors together with occlusal mirrors (**Figure 7**).

They can also be used easily with contrastors (**Figures 8** and **9**).

Columbia retractors

These double-ended cheek retractors can be used in pairs to retract either upper or lower lips for occlusal views (**Figures 10** and **11**).

Similarly, split or half retractors can also be equally useful (**Figure 12**).

There are several single-handed retractors available for occlusal views; some are in the form of contrastors (**Figures 13** to **18**).

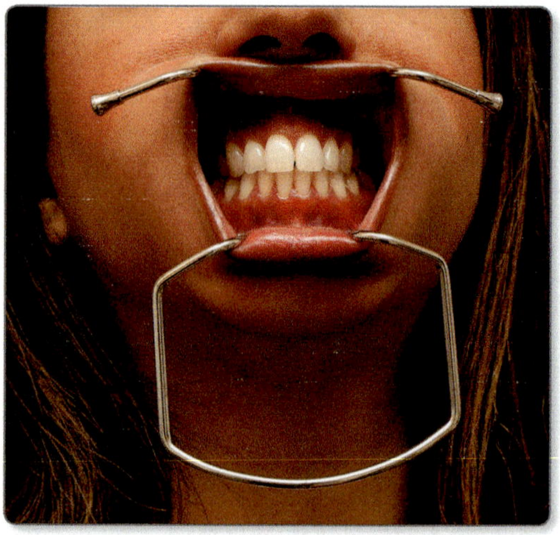

Figure 7 Oringer retractor.
(*Courtesy:* Dr Neel Jaiswal)

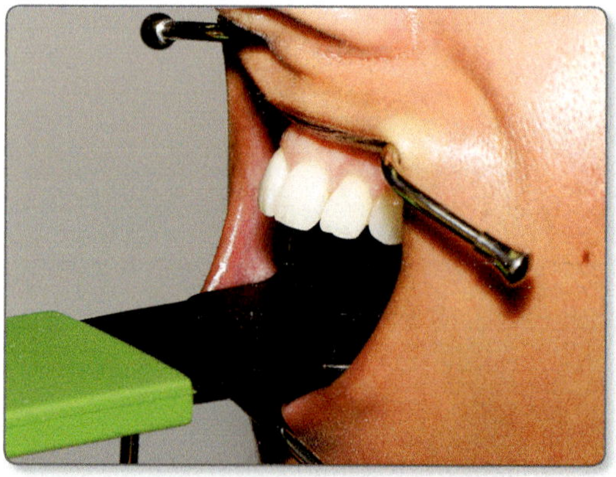

Figure 8 Doctorseyes contrastor in combination with oringer retractor.

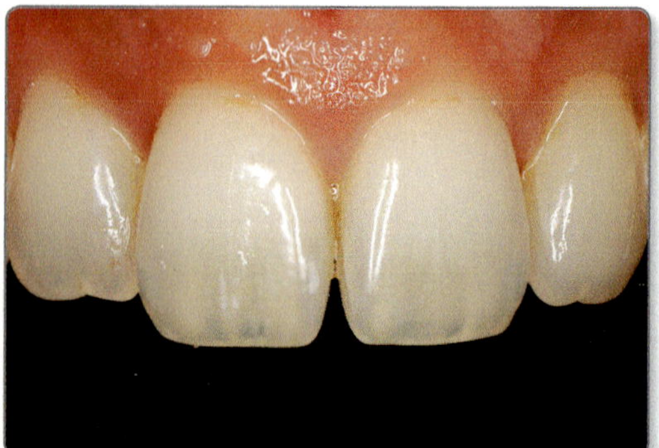

Figure 9 Image with contrastor *in situ.*
(*Courtesy:* Dr Neel Jaiswal)

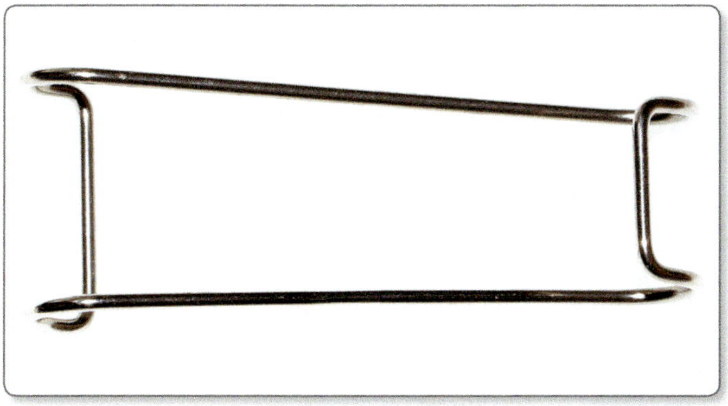

Figure 10 Columbia retractor.

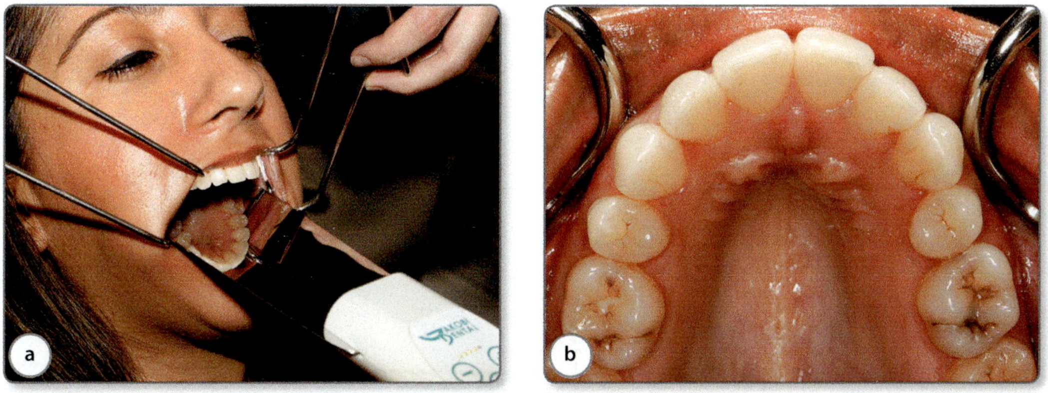

Figure 11 (a) Columbia retractors + Jakobi de-misting mirror; (b) Image using set-up as (a). [*Courtesy*: Dr Neel Jaiswal, (b)]

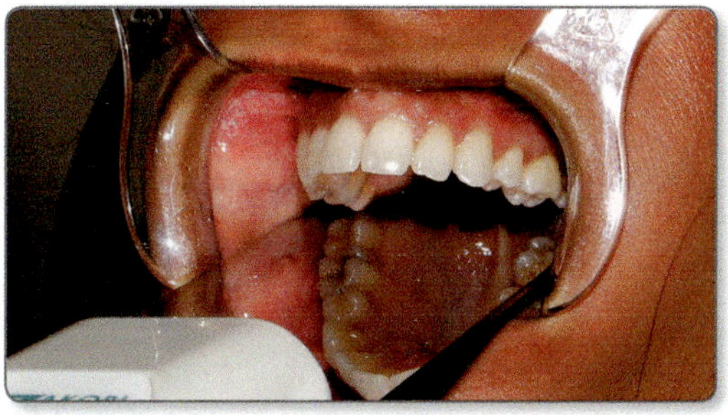

Figure 12 Cut down retractors.

Mirrors

Mirrors must have the reflective coating on the surface to avoid a ghost image from the mirror surface when the actual reflective material is on the back. The average make-up mirror being a typical example.

Figure 19 shows the subject in contact with a mirror with a rear surface reflective coating and a ghost image from the surface. **Figure 20** shows the subject in contact with a front surface mirror.

Mirrors available for dental photography are generally either chrome plated or titanium plated (**Figures 21** and **22**). Doctorseyes also manufacture models under the 'ultra-bright' label (**Figure 23**). One of the advantages claimed for the more expensive mirrors is an increase in reflectivity. This advantage has been negated by 'through-the-lens' (TTL) flash metering, which will automatically compensate for any reduction or increase in the light intensity. However, the coating can affect the accuracy of the image colour when the mirror is placed in direct contact with the subject.

The full-arch images (**Figures 21** to **23**) show very little difference and are totally acceptable. However, when the same mirrors are placed in contact with the subject, the differences are quite significant.

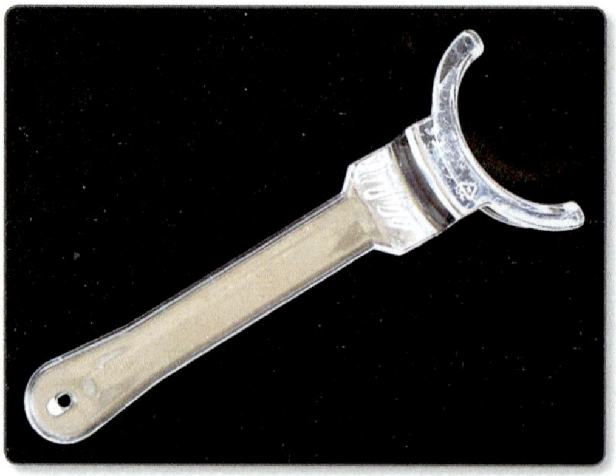

Figure 13 Plastic occlusal retractor.

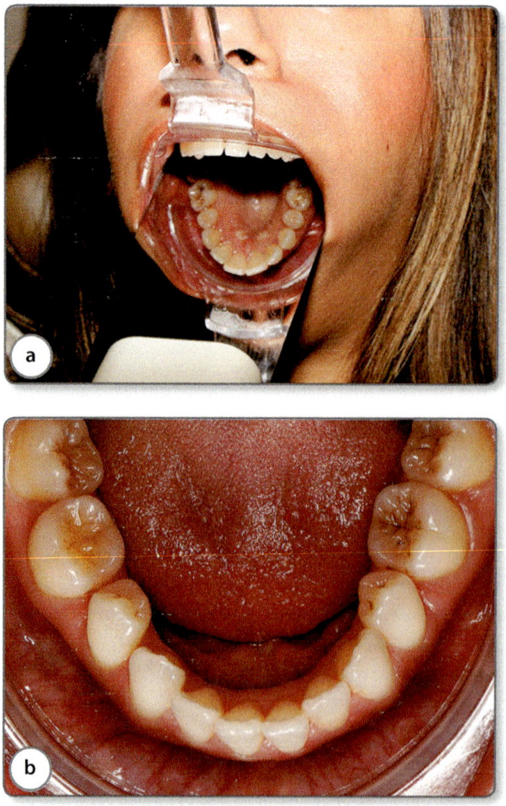

Figures 14a and b Images using plastic lip retractor.
(*Courtesy:* Dr Neel Jaiswal)

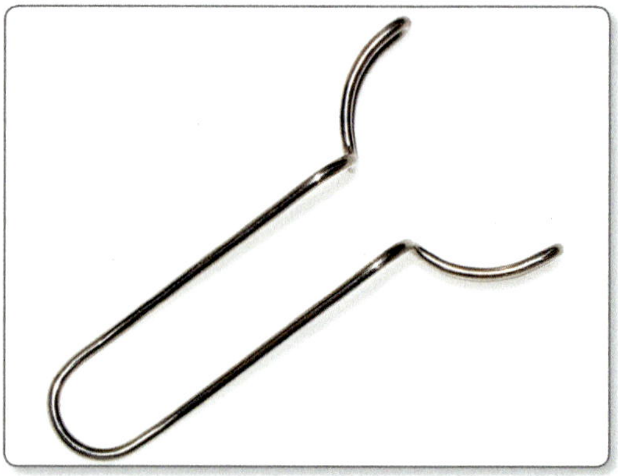

Figure 15 Jakobi vestibular retractor CRLAF version.

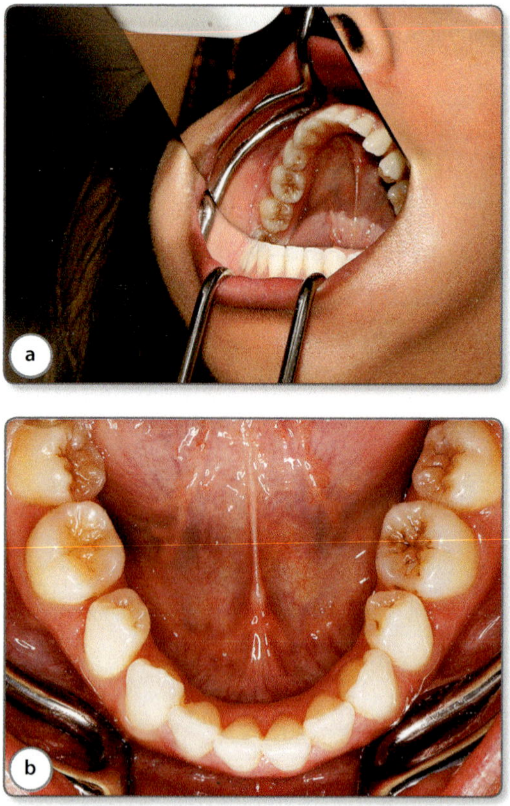

Figures 16a and b Images using Jakobi vestibular retractor CRLAF version.
(*Courtesy:* Dr Neel Jaiswal)

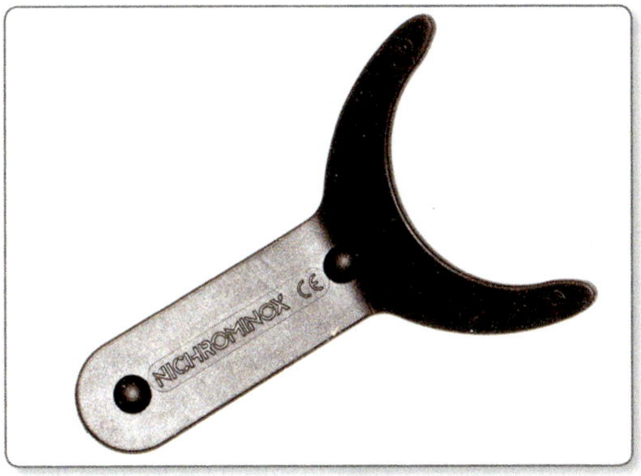

Figure 17 Nichrominox retractor/contrastor.

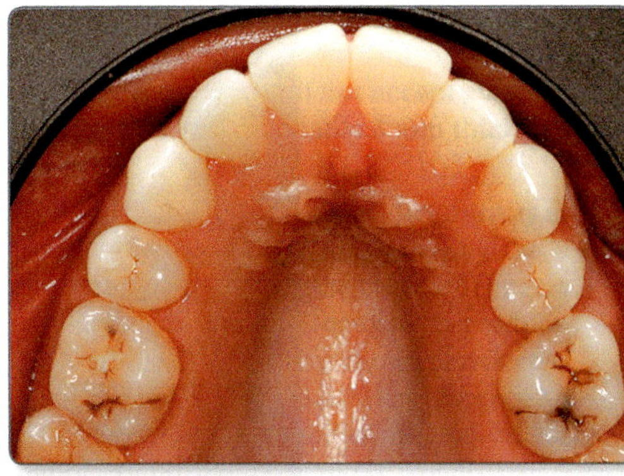

Figure 18 Image using Nichrominox contrastor/retractor. (*Courtesy:* Dr Neel Jaiswal)

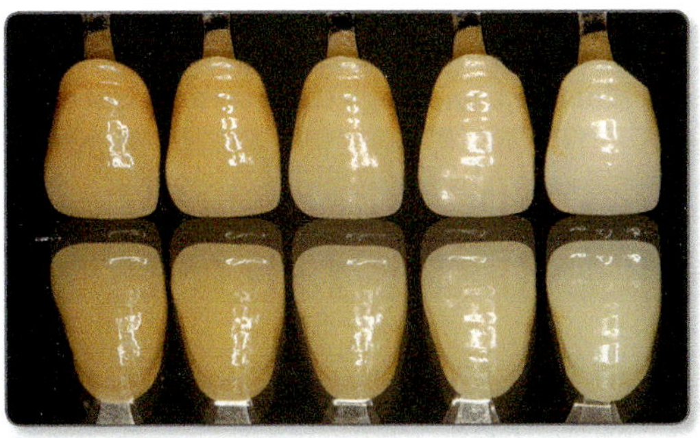

Figure 19 The subject in contact with a mirror with a rear surface reflective coating and a ghost image from the surface.

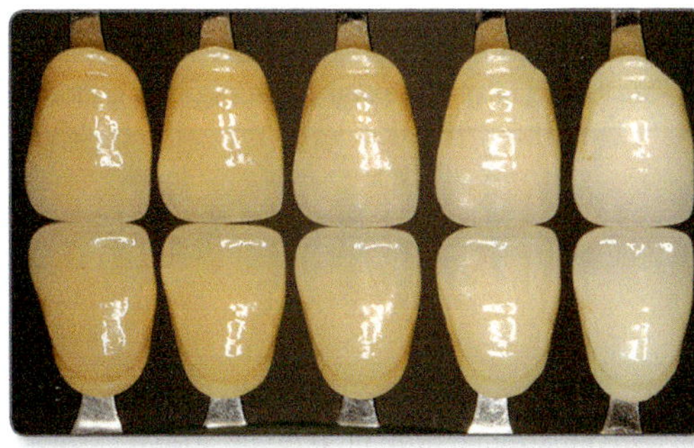

Figure 20 The subject in contact with a front surface mirror.

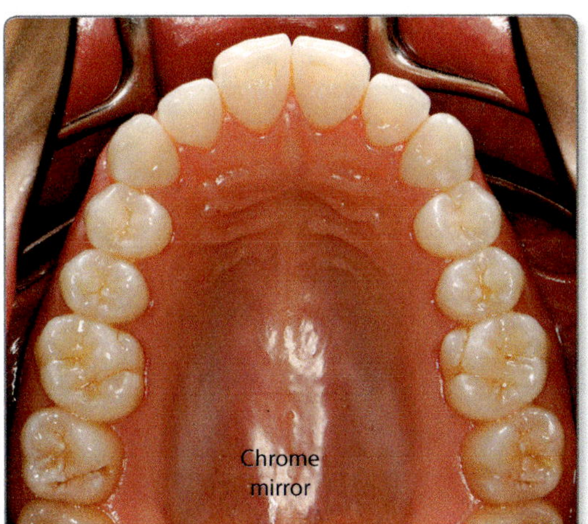

Figure 21 Image in chrome mirror.

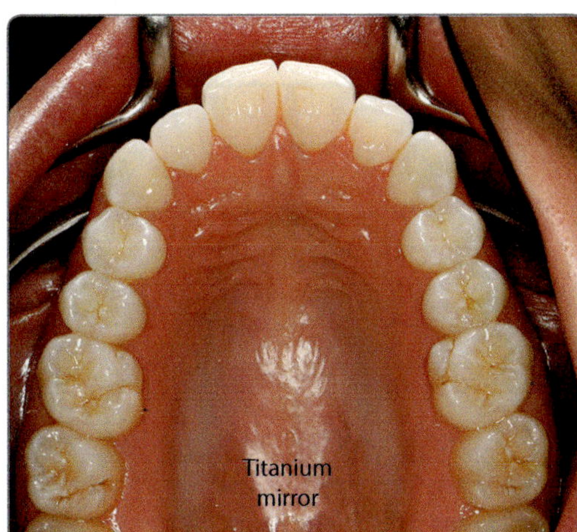

Figure 22 Image in titanium mirror.

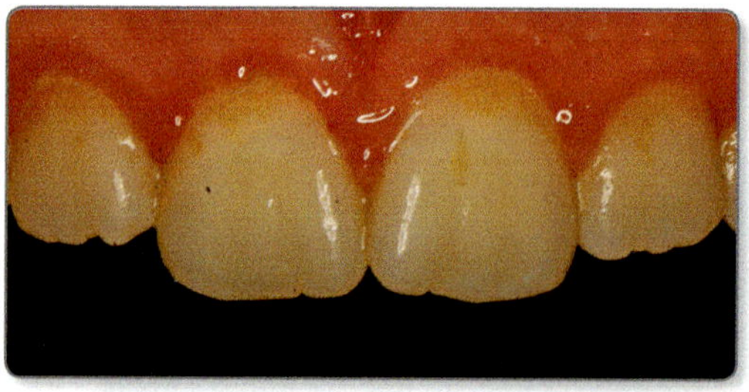

Figure 37 Image using T10 flash direct.

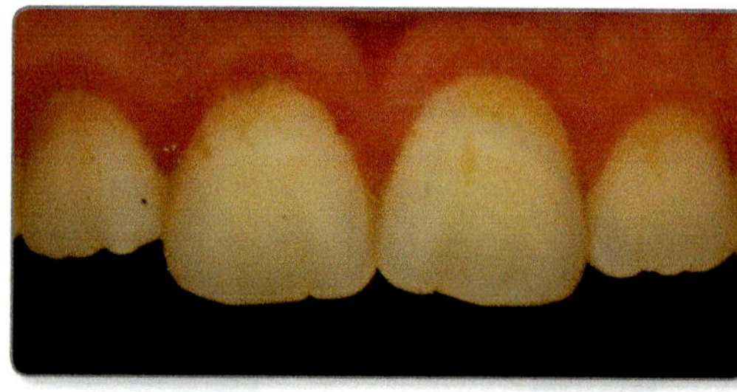

Figure 38 Image using T10 with polarising filter.

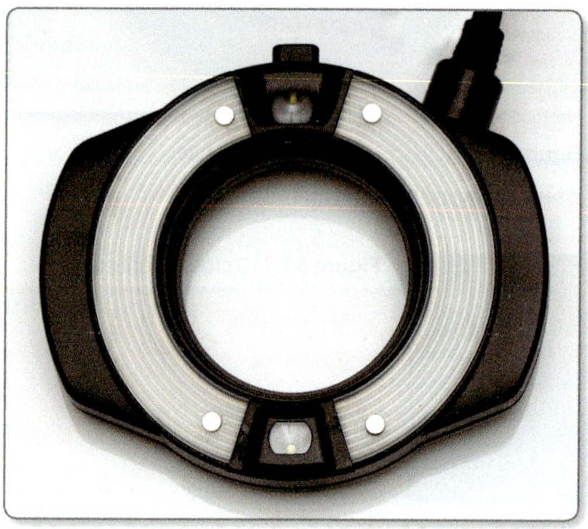

Figure 39 Canon MR EX II flash etc. flash with magnets.

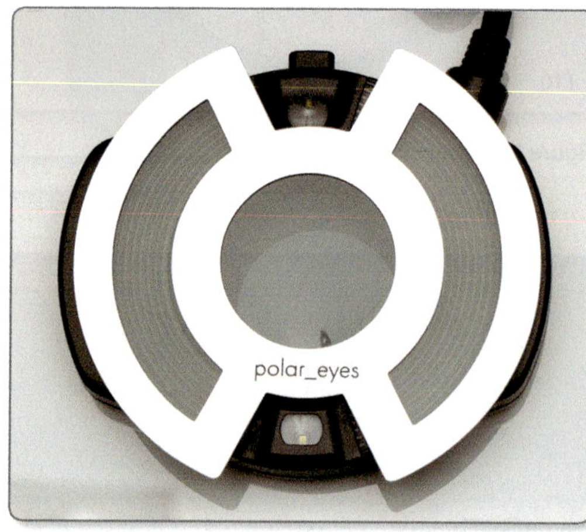

Figure 40 The polar_eyes filter attached.

Scale

Photographs of lesions should always be taken against a scale (**Figures 41** and **42**). Small stainless steel rulers or a forensic scale are ideal (**Figure 43**).

Safety

Many colleagues take some images from above and behind a supine patient; the author advises the use of either the neck strap supplied with the camera or a wrist strap such as the 'clutch' (**Figure 44**).

Clinical outfits tend to be heavy and occasionally are required to be used one handed. A pistol grip can be very useful in this respect, but compatibility with one's camera will need checking (**Figure 45**).

If weight of the outfit is a serious issue, the following information might be of interest.

Camera bodies

Current entry level bodies such as the Canon 250D and Nikon D5600 will do everything and more than is required for clinical work. Being mainly of polycarbonate construction, at around 450 g (16 oz), they are half the weight of their metal-based higher specified models.

Lenses

Without exception, all the lenses mentioned have a maximum aperture of f2.8. Thus, in theory, they all have the same specification with respect to their focal lengths. However, there is quite a variation in cost, which poses the question – is a lens costing £2X twice as

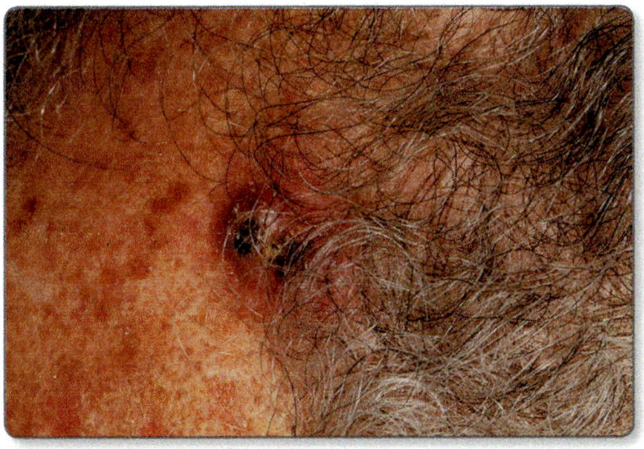

Figure 41 Squamous cell carcinoma.

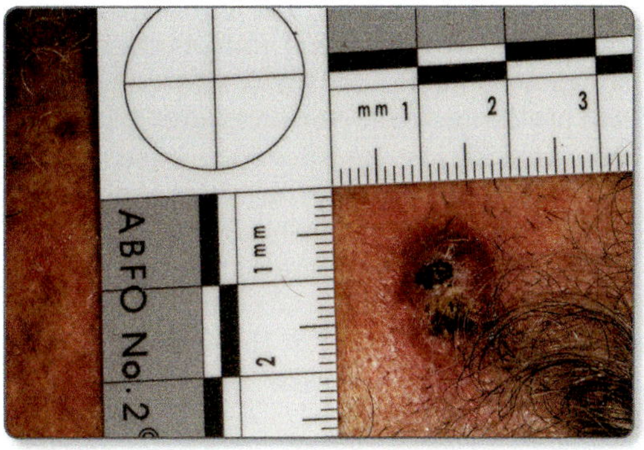

Figure 42 Forensic scale.

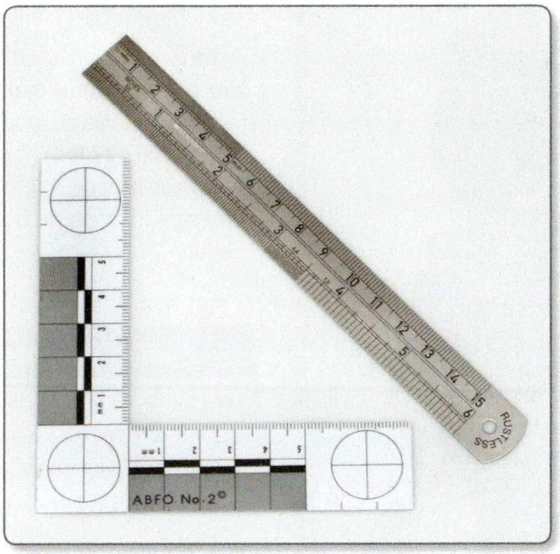

Figure 43 Forensic and normal rulers.

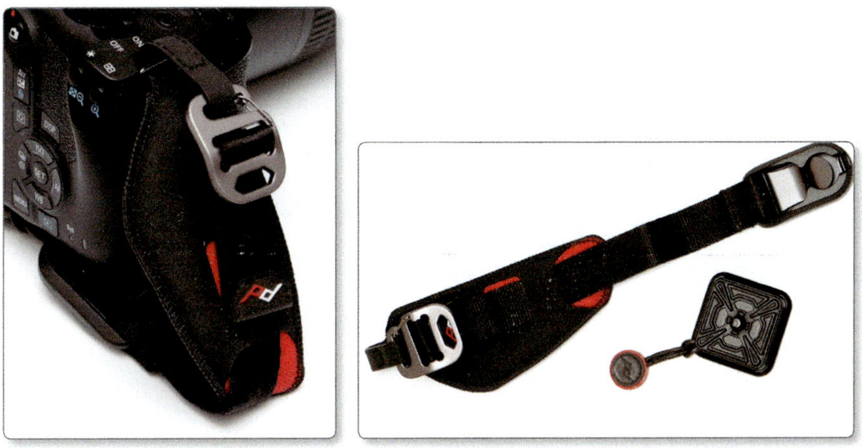

Figure 44 Clutch wrist strap.

good as a lens costing £X? The more expensive lenses will have more metal and less plastic in their construction and are designed for hard professional use. Not necessarily a major consideration in a dental practice. Therefore, their optical performance would be the major factor. Probably the distinguishing feature separating the cheapest from the most expensive would be the lens' performance at its widest aperture, i.e., f2.8. However, in dental photography, this aperture is virtually never used and in the context of quality required for clinical work, all those described would be totally adequate. What may be of interest and considered with the other components is that of weight and bulk (**Table 1** and **Figure 46**).

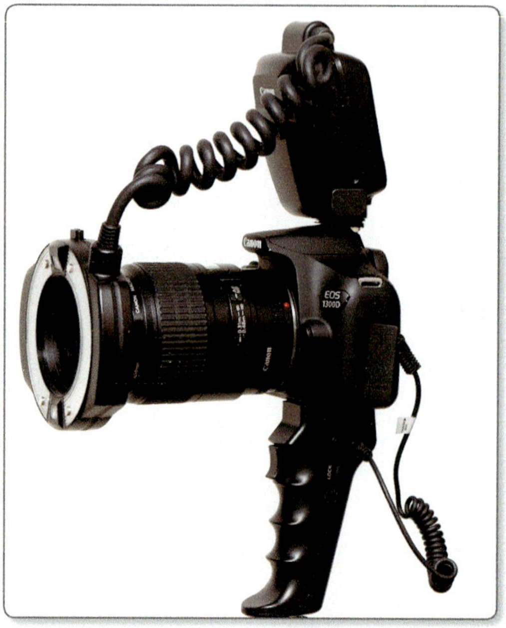

Figure 45 Camera mounted on pistol grip.

Flash systems

The Canon MR 14 EX-II and Nissin MF-18 are 450 g (16 oz); the Canon MT 26 is of 600 g (21 oz). The lightweights are the Metz MS-1 weighs in at 160 g (5.6 oz) and the Lester Dine Ring/point unit weighs at 286 g (10 oz). Note the Lester Dine unit is available for Nikon and Canon only and Metz MS-1 compatibility with TTL metering must be checked prior to purchase (see Chapter 3).

Thus, a hybrid outfit of entry level body, Tamron 90 mm un-stabilised lens and Metz MS-1 flash, would weigh at around 1,000 g (2 lbs) and at least 450 g (1 lbs) lighter than a regular Canon/Nikon set-up and 1,000 g (2 lbs) lighter than a camera with a metal body.

Table1 Weights of different lenses.

Lens	Ounces	Grams
1. CANON 100 mm stabilised	22.1	626
2. CANON 100 mm non-stabilised	21.2	600
3. NIKON 105 mm stabilised	27.9	791
4. SIGMA 105 mm stabilised	25.6	726
5. TAMRON 90 mm stabilised	21.5	610
6. TAMRON 90 mm non-stabilised	14.3	404

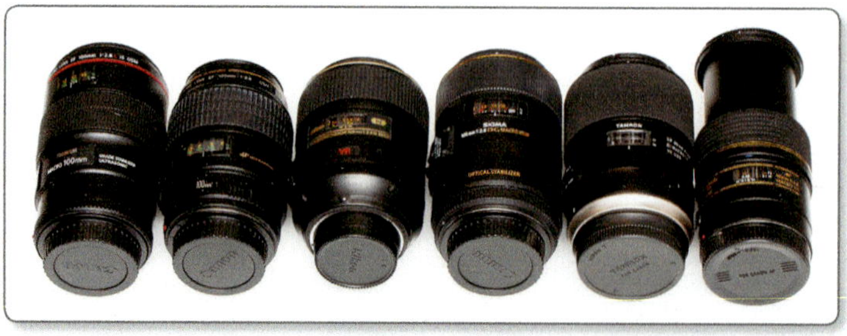

Figure 46 Lenses in the same order as shown in Table 1.

7 Comparison of lighting systems on teeth and models

Introduction

This section sets out to compare smiles captured with different lighting set-ups. A typical set-up is shown at **Figure 1**. All the original images were of a full smile (see **Figure 2**), but the comparative images have been cropped to save space. By pre-setting 1:3 on the magnification scale on 90 mm, 100 mm, and 105 mm macro lenses and moving the camera assembly to achieve focus, a commissure to commissure image can be consistently achieved (see **Figure 2**). On most macro lenses this scale is in yellow/orange.

Reflections from teeth will depend on the light source and angles of illumination. The aim of this chapter is to investigate many of the options and hopefully assist the operator in his or her choice of equipment. **Figure 2** could be considered as typical taken with any 'ring' flash with the flash units placed at 9 and 3 o'clock. The glare will increase if closer views are taken (see **Figure 3**), and if more aesthetic images are required of single teeth, it is worth considering cropping the full smile view (see **Figure 4**).

System comparison

Whilst some glare might be considered intrusive and potentially mask minor pathology, an image without highlights could be considered flat and not life-like. **Figure 5** was taken using large studio soft boxes at some distance from the subject, whereas **Figure 6** shows the same subject using typical on camera 'ring-flash.' Note that studio lighting does not illuminate the buccal corridor.

The following images show a direct comparison using the Canon MR EX II 'ring' flash (**Figure 7** and **8a** and **b**) and the Canon MT24/26 twin light system (**Figures 9** and **10**). The simple expedient of placing the flash units at 11 and 1 o'clock has reduced the impact of the highlights and increased the incisal translucency (**Figures 11** to **14**).

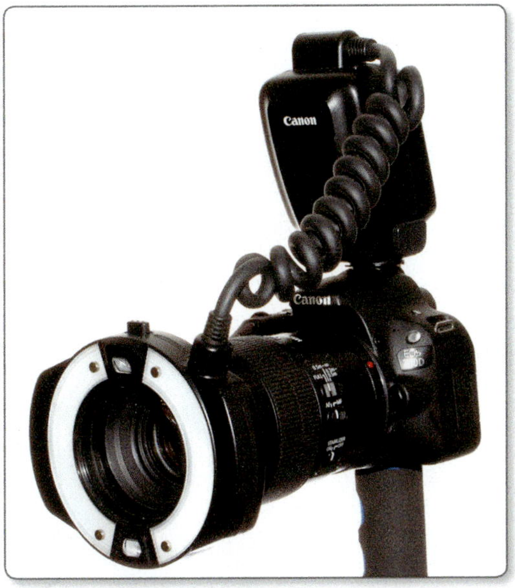

Figure 1 Canon MR 14 EX II 'ring' flash.

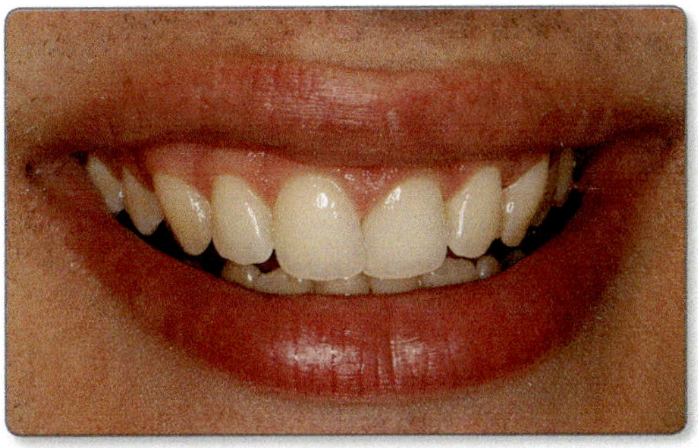

Figure 2 Image taken using standard ring flash set-up as Figure 1. Magnification ratio on 100 mm lens set at 1:3.

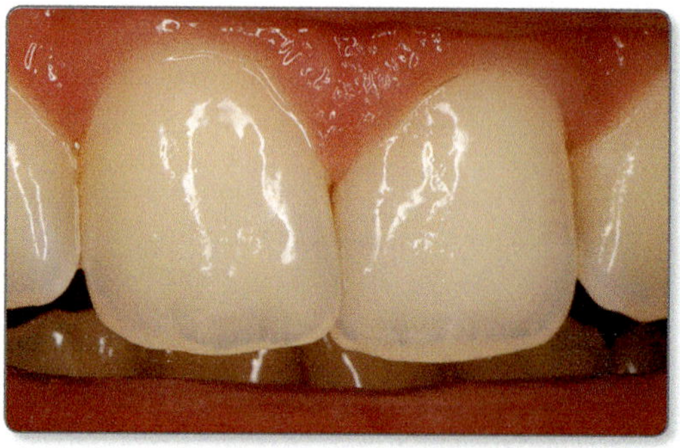

Figure 3 Image taken @ 1:1.

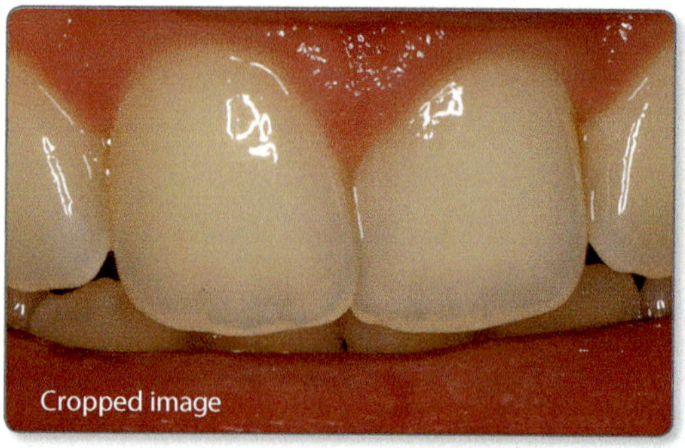

Figure 4 Image at Figure 2 cropped.

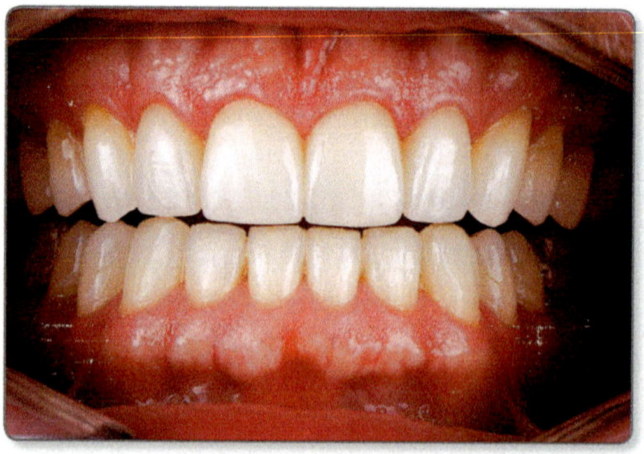

Figure 5 Taken using studio flash. Two large soft boxes above and behind patient.
(*Courtesy:* Dr Shameek Popat)

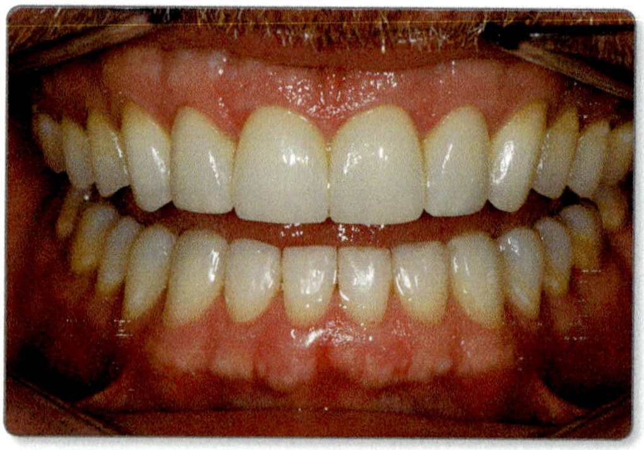

Figure 6 Taken using Metz MS-1 flash.
(*Courtesy:* Dr Shameek Popat)

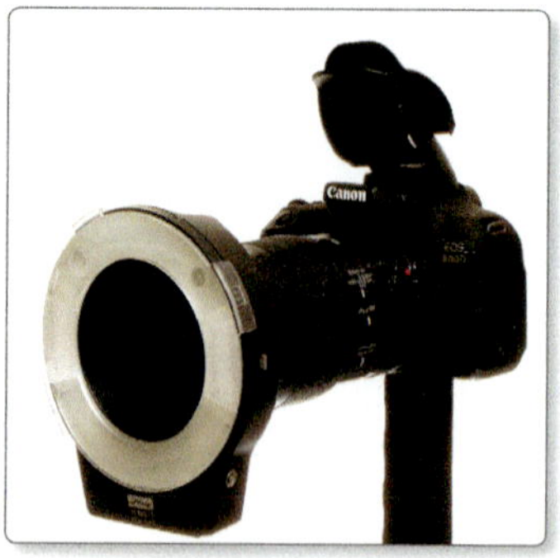

Figure 7 Camera set-up for Figure 6.
(*Courtesy:* Dr Shameek Popat)

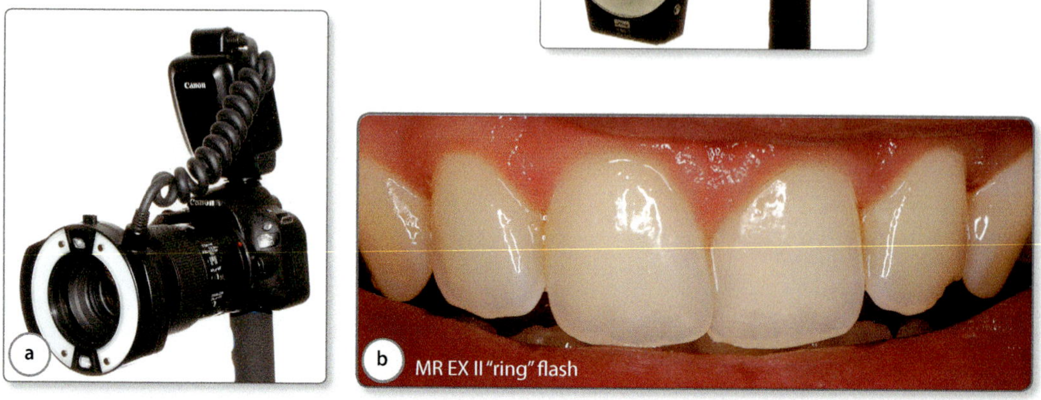

Figure 8 Canon MR 14 EX II flash. Using set up as shown in Figure (a).

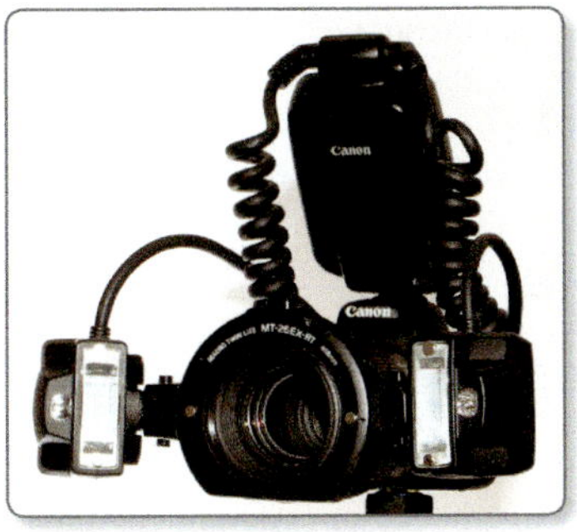

Figure 9 Canon MT 24 flash.

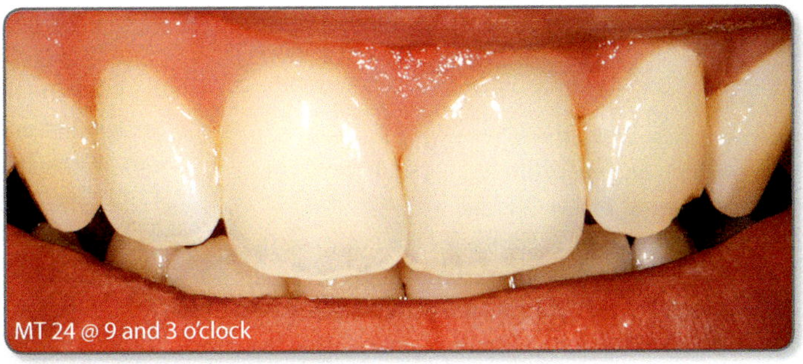

Figure 10 Image taken with MT 24 flash units @ 9 and 3 o'clock.

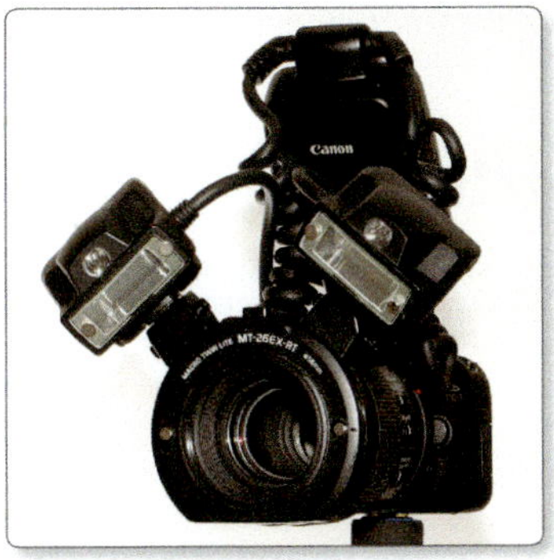

Figure 11 Canon MT 24/26 flash @ 11 and 1 o'clock.

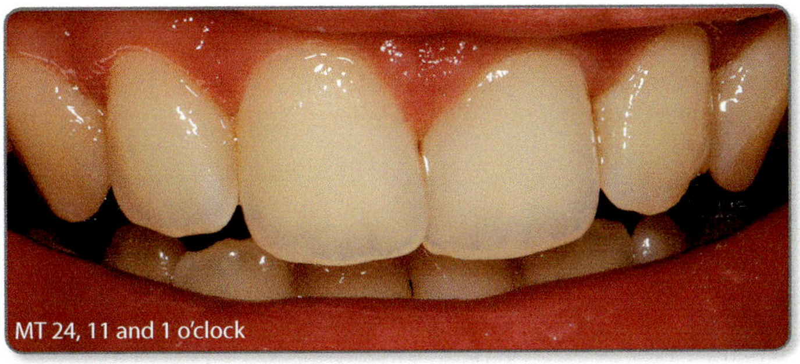

Figure 12 Image taken with MT 24 flash units @ 11 and 1 o'clock.

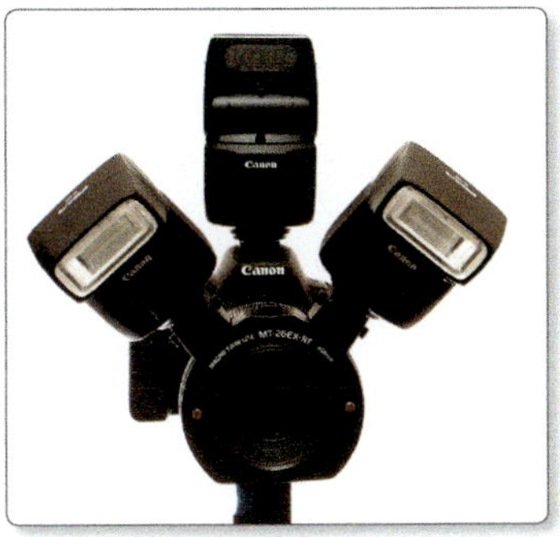

Figure 13 Two Canon EL 100 flash units on MT 24/26 mount.

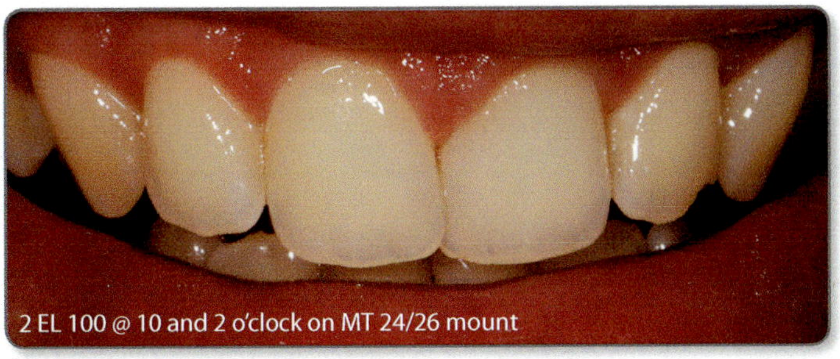

Figure 14 Image taken with 2 EL 100 units @ 10 and 2 o'clock.

Bracket systems

Axis

The Axis bracket is supplied with interchangeable arms which accept either Nikon SB R200 flash units or Canon MT24/26 flashes easily. The author managed to fit Canon EL 100 units with slight difficulty but no third party flashes. It is the simplest of all the bracket systems fixing the units at 45° to the optical axis. By increasing the flash to subject distance the glare is reduced in comparison to other typical 'on camera' flash units (**Figures 15** to **18**).

Note that any system that places the flash heads above the optical axis, will produce shadowing from the upper lip and increase incisal translucency.

All the other bracket systems are far more versatile in allowing a wider choice of flash systems plus any other accessories such as soft boxes and bouncers.

PhotoMed, Owl, Agnos, and Molaris brackets

All these brackets enable the operator to place flash units at various distances from the lens either on, or in many instances, above the lens axis. They enable a wider choice of flash systems which can either be used alone or in combination with other accessories such as soft boxes and bouncers. The standard 'Twin Systems' from Canon and Nikon utilise very small flash heads, MT 24/26, and SB R200, respectively, neither system will allow the easy use of small soft boxes or bouncers. Canon make a small flash unit, the EL 100 and the Nissin i40 is available in Canon and Nikon formats. Both systems can be wirelessly triggered, the Canon by an additional EL 100 or Metz 400 flash.

All the brackets allow close approximation of the flash heads to the lens and this will give a similar result to the 'standard' ring flash.

Boxes and bouncers

Lumiquest, make a selection of flash accessories easily attached or removed using Velcro straps (**Figures 19** to **21**).

The bouncers and ultrasoft units reflect the flash towards the subject, the mini soft box softens and diffuses a direct source (**Figures 22** to **27**).

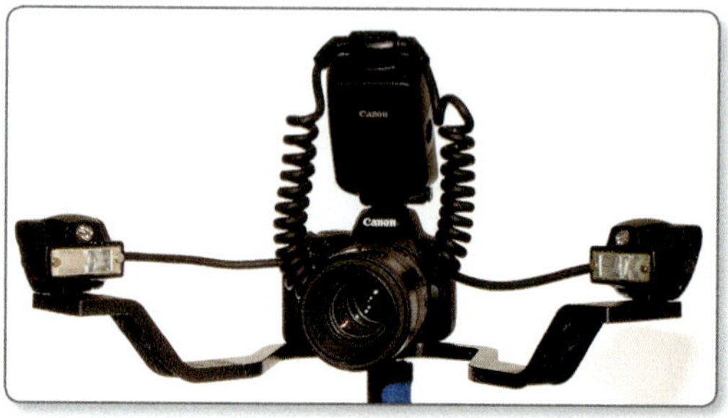

Figure 15 Canon MT 24 flash units on Axis bracket.

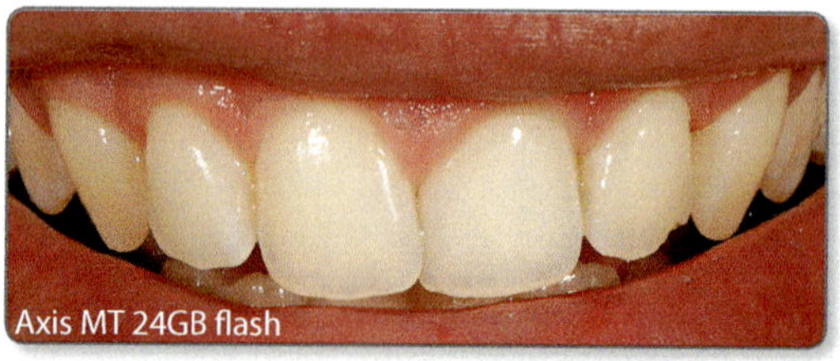

Figure 16 Image taken using MT 24 on Axis bracket.

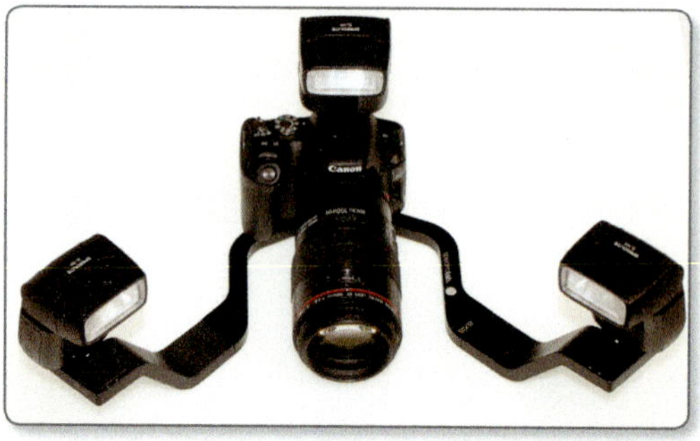

Figure 17 Two Canon EL 100 flash units on Axis bracket with third EL 100 as trigger.

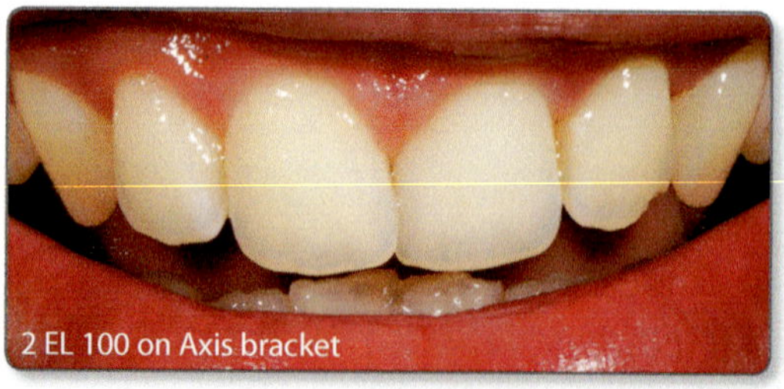

Figure 18 Image taken using EL 100 flash units on Axis bracket.

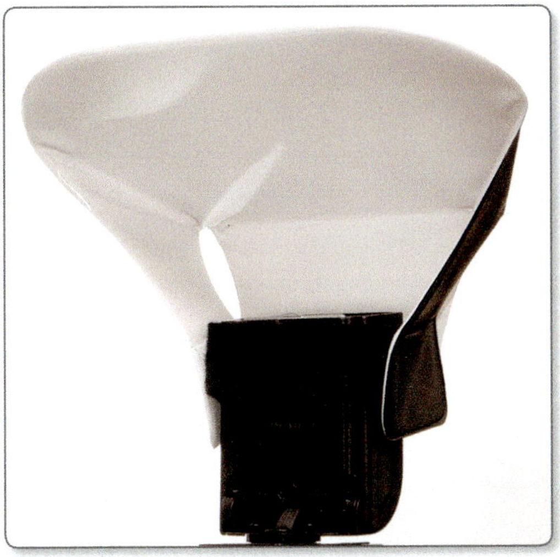

Figure 19 Lumiquest bouncer.

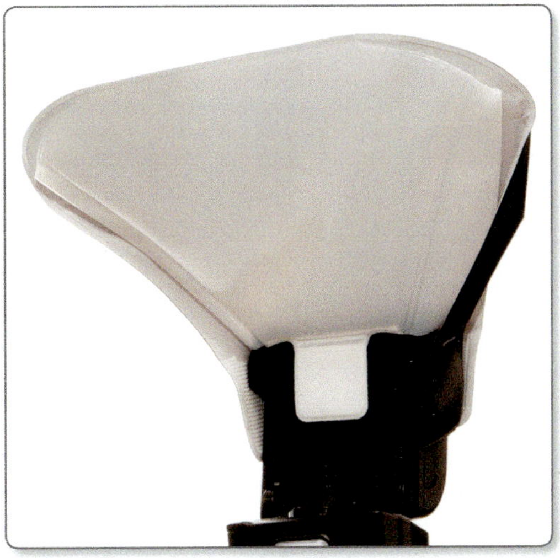

Figure 20 Lumiquest ultrasoft.

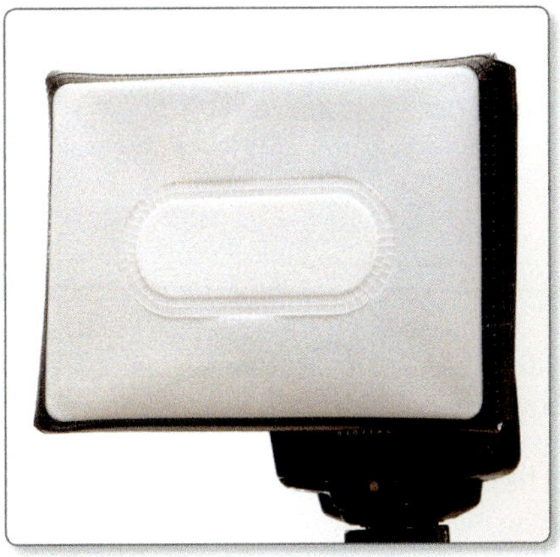

Figure 21 Lumiquest mini soft box.

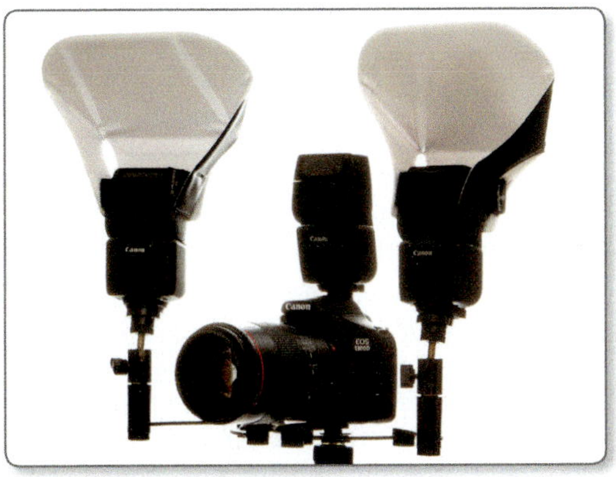

Figure 22 Two EL 100 flash units + bouncers @ 10 and 2 o'clock (Owl).

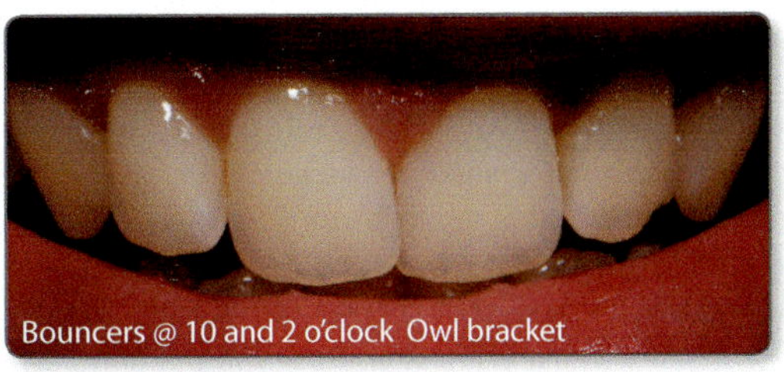

Figure 23 Image taken with bouncer as set-up in Figure 22.

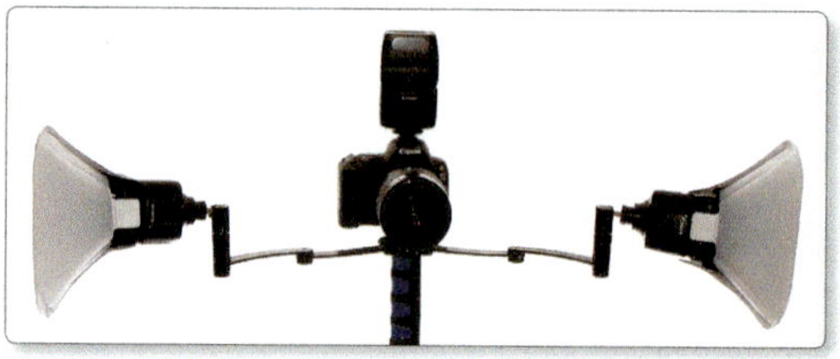

Figure 24 Two EL 100 flash units + ultrasoft bouncers @ maximum distance from lens (Owl).

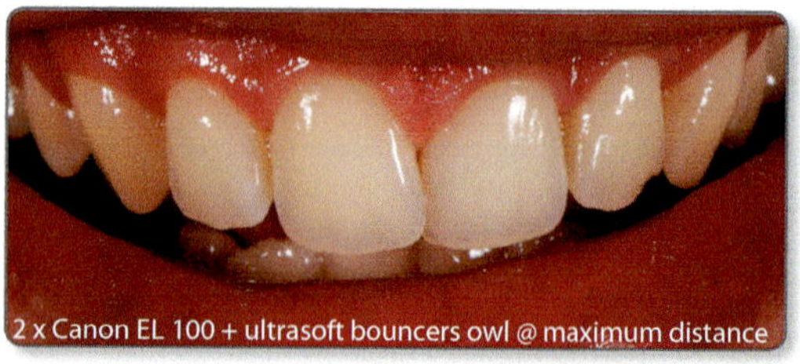

Figure 25 Image using set-up as shown in Figure 24.

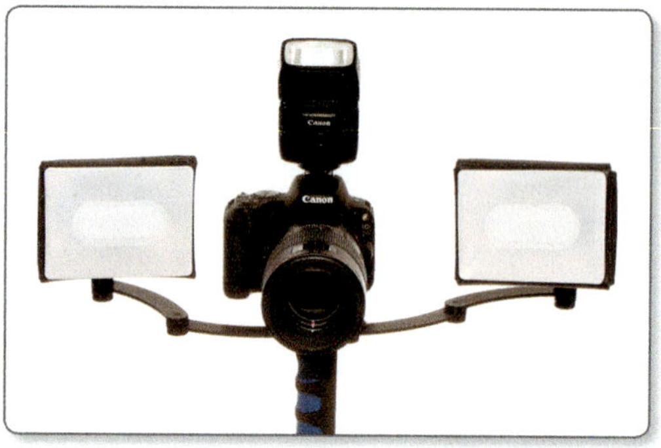

Figure 26 Two El 100 flash units + mini soft boxes close to the lens.

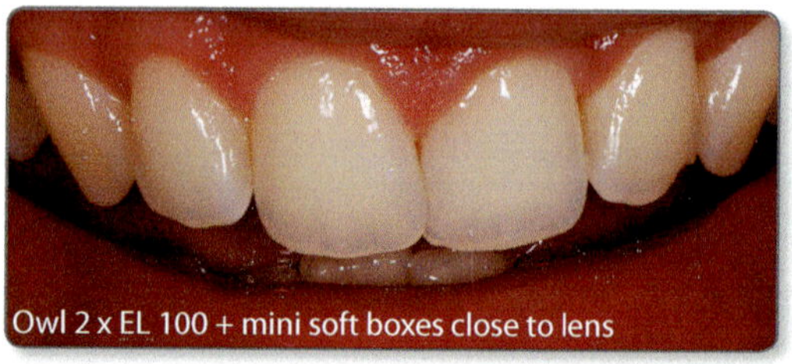

Figure 27 Image using set-up as shown in Figure 26.

Studio lighting

The minimum requirement for studio lighting is usually two soft boxes placed above and behind the camera. They offer continuous lighting for modelling purposes, but built-in flashes triggered wirelessly by the camera are used to illuminate the subject (see **Figures 28** and **29**).

Alternatively, more compact studio systems are available from Rotolight and Essential Photos. The NEO 2 (Rotolight) incorporates LED continuous lighting plus an internal flash which can be triggered by the camera (**Figure 30**). The main advantage of continuous lighting is the ability to see the effect of shadowing, see **Figure 31**. This image was taken with a single handheld Rotolight NEO 2 near the subject and without using the flash. The flash function can be operated by a PC cable for a single unit, or multiple units by using an appropriate wireless trigger, e.g. the EL-Skyport. The individual units can be battery (6 AA cells) or mains powered.

Figure 32 was taken in a studio situation with two NEO 2 units illuminating the subject and one used to eliminate background shadow.

Figure 33 shows similar unilateral lighting on the face but by using a black velvet background the rear shadow is eliminated. The use of a light panel would achieve a similar shadow-less background. In this instance the flash function was utilised.

Essential photos produce a large LED ring light, the Pixapro RICO240 (see **Figures 34** and **35**).

Setting up a single lighting unit

Pixapro RICO240

This lighting unit can be mounted on a purpose made stand or on a tripod placed in front of the camera. For the latter you may need to purchase a spigot (**Figure 36**) to mount the light securely.

The LEDs are balanced for daylight therefore the white balance (WB) setting on the camera should be entered accordingly. Compared with electronic flash these units are not very powerful and to utilise a shutter speed of around 1/200 sec. and aperture of f4, the author recommends an ISO of 1600. The images in this section were all taken at those settings. If considering such a system, the

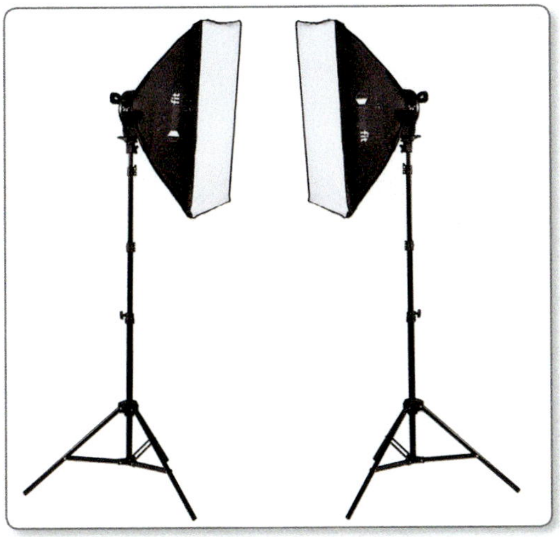

Figure 28 Typical studio set-up.

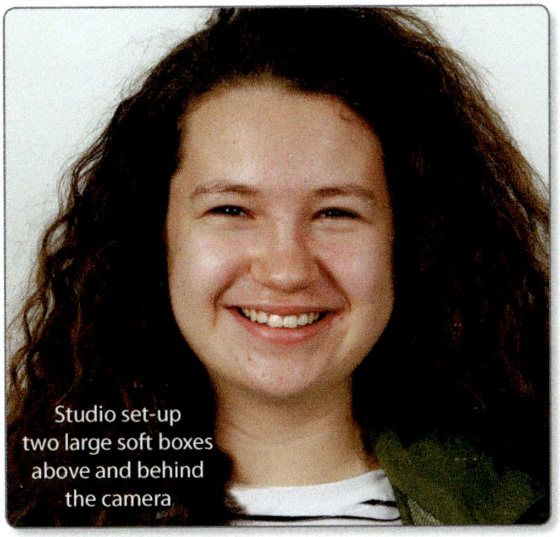
Studio set-up
two large soft boxes
above and behind
the camera

Figure 29 Image using studio flash (Knight dental design).

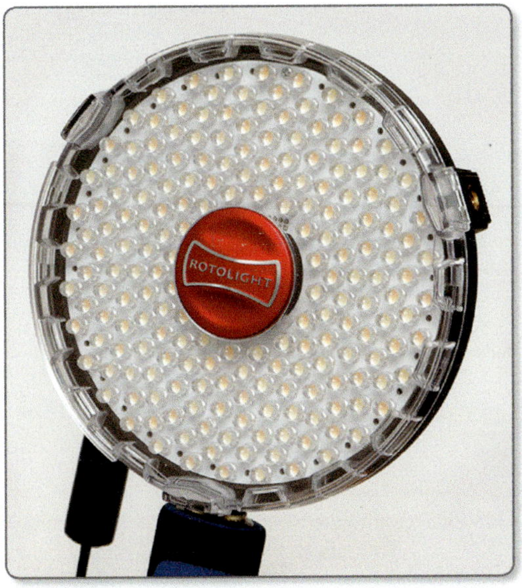
ROTOLIGHT

Figure 30 Rotolight NEO 2 light unit.

more expensive optically stabilised lenses would be advantageous.

NEO 2 led light

Two or more units can be placed on stands or a single unit placed in the camera's hot shoe. In this case the Rotolight hot shoe/PC lead adapter will be required to trigger the flash (see **Figure 37**), and an adaptor (see **Figure 38**), to mount the light onto the shoe. Whilst the NEO 2 is quite intense, the inbuilt flash is required to boost the illumination when using a single unit mounted on the camera (**Figure 39**).

Figures 40 and **41** were taken against a white wall using single lighting units. **Figure 35** showing the Pixapro RICO240; **Figure 40** showing

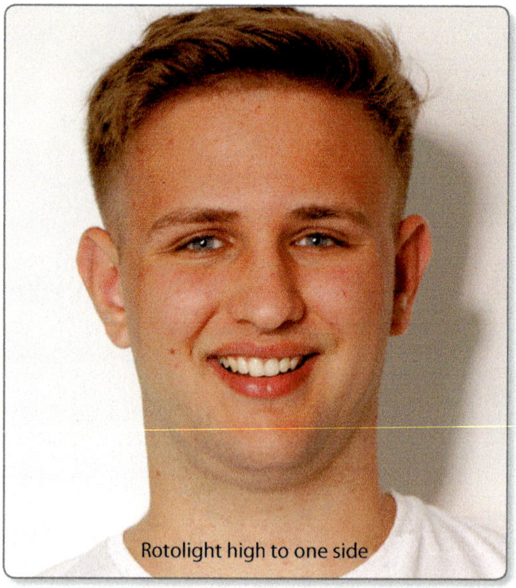

Figure 31 Taken with single NEO 2.

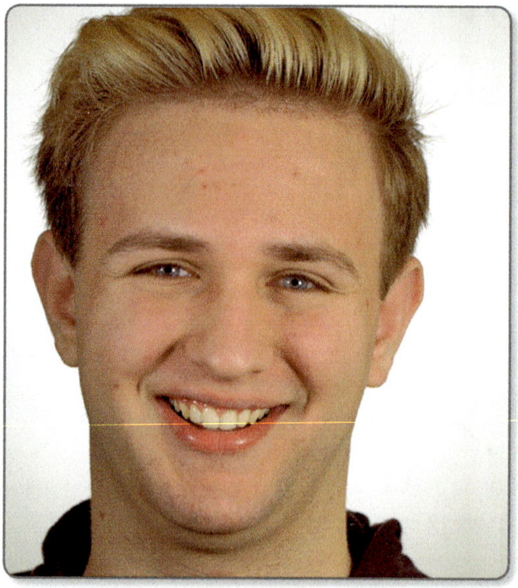

Figure 32 Taken with NEO 2 in studio. Two lights on subject and third eliminating background shadow. (*Courtesy:* Rotolight)

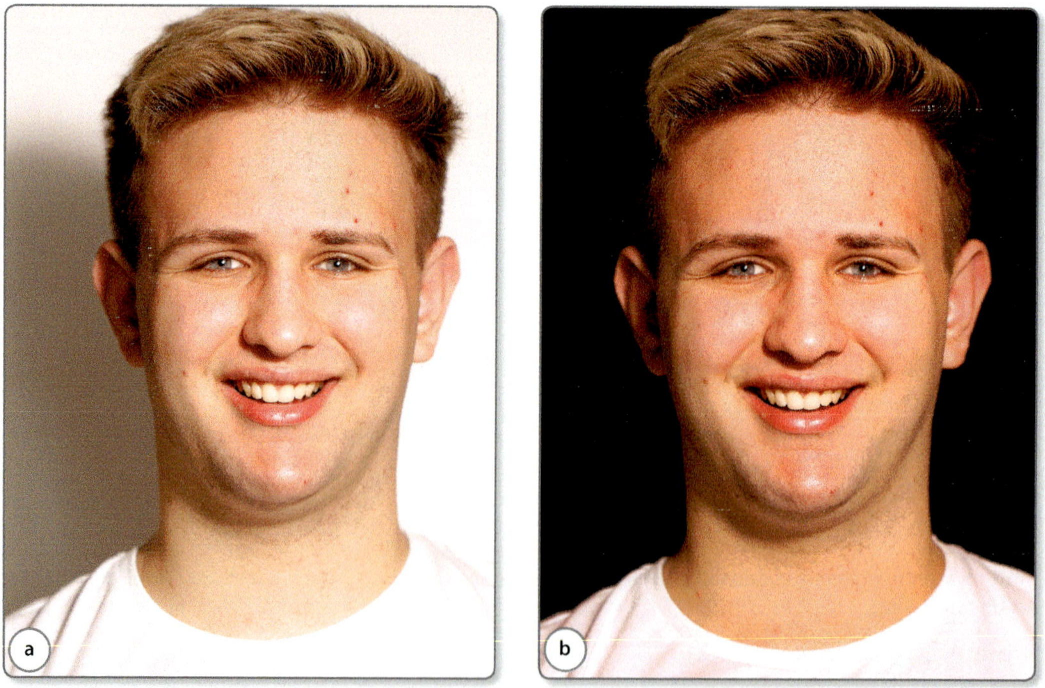

Figures 33a and b Images taken with unilateral NEO 2 + internal flash.

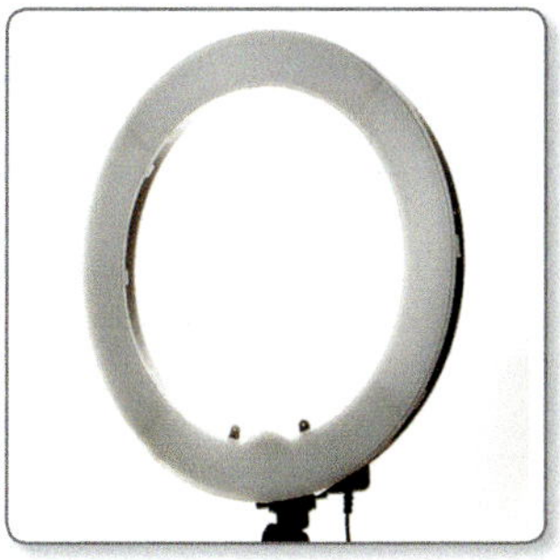

Figure 34 Pixapro RICO 240 LED ringlight.

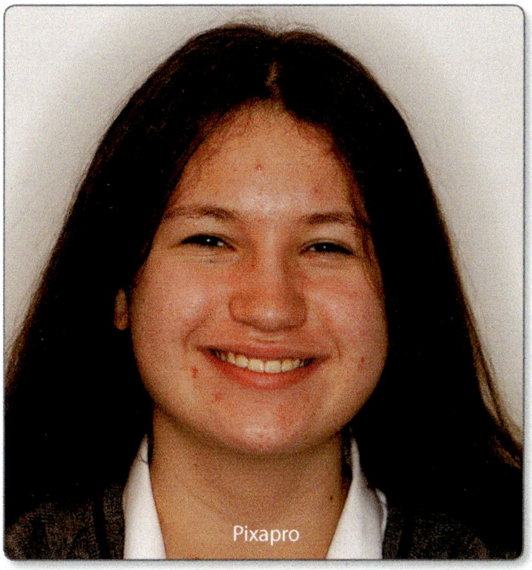

Figure 35 Pixapro RICO240.

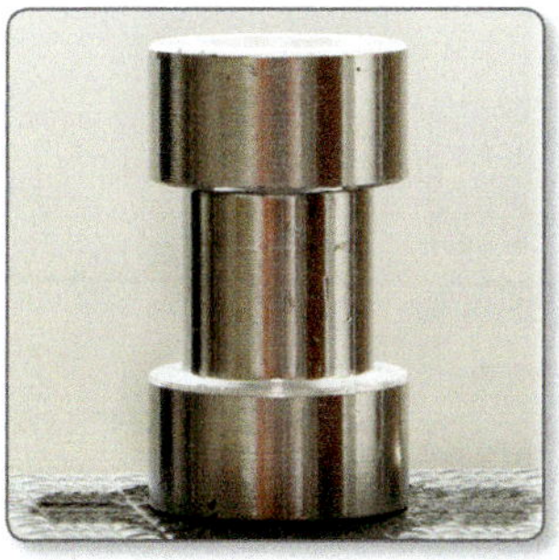

Figure 36 Spigot to attach Pixapro ringlight to a tripod.

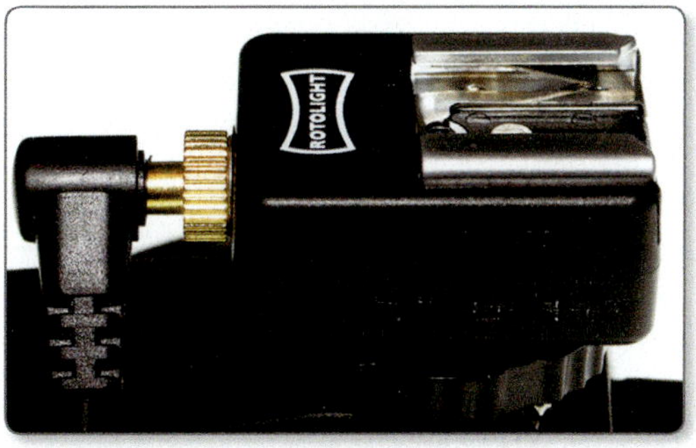

Figure 37 Hot shoe PC cord adaptor.

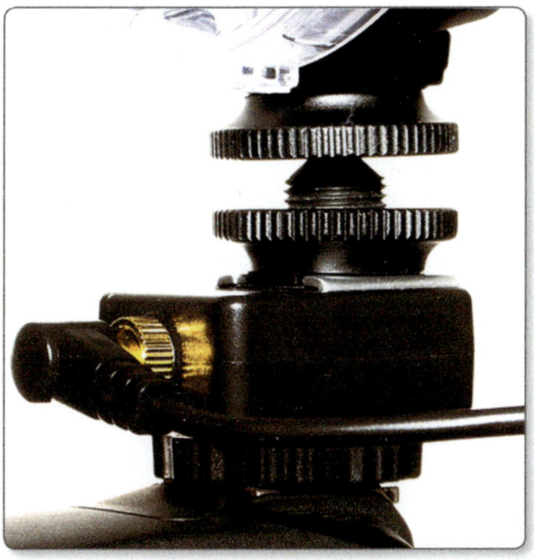

Figure 38 Hot shoe to NEO 2 adaptor.

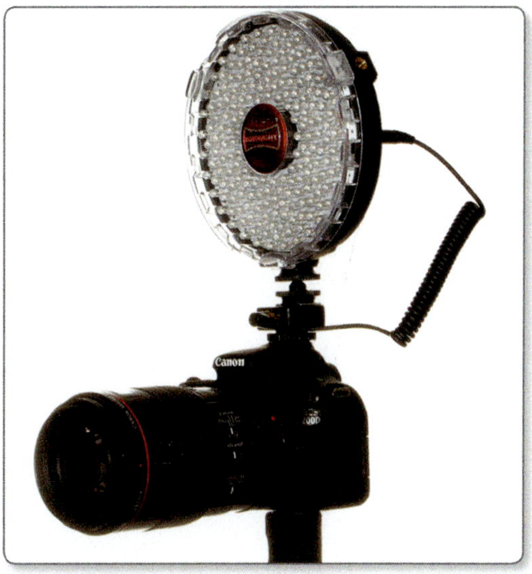

Figure 39 Camera with NEO 2 attached.

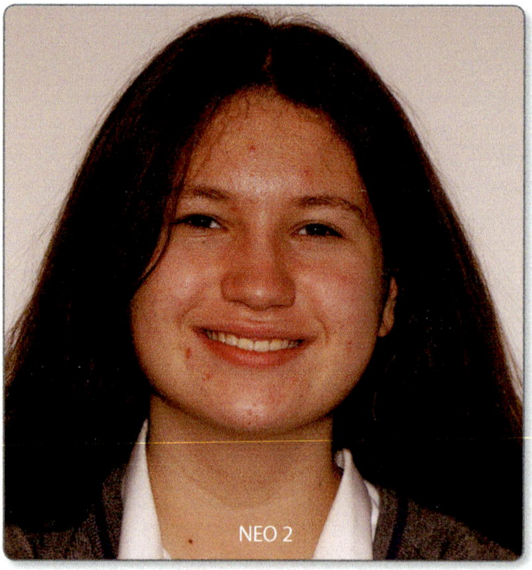

Figure 40 NEO 2 set-up as shown in Figure 39.

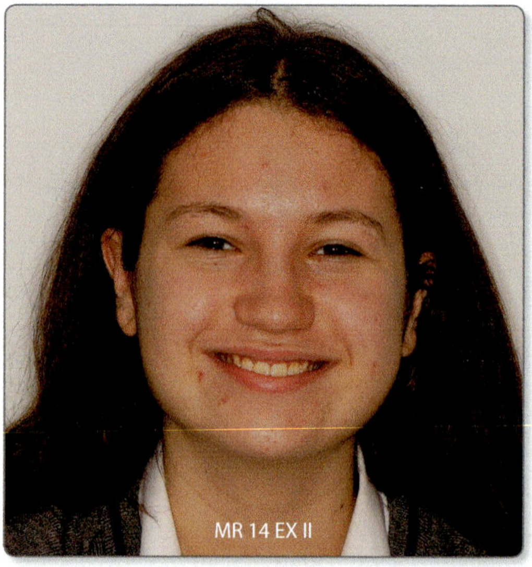

Figure 41 MR EX II flash. Using set up as shown in Figure 1.

a camera mounted NEO 2 plus the inbuilt flash (see **Figure 39**); and **Figure 41** showing the standard set up with the Canon MR 14 EX II ring flash.

Unfortunately, one cannot just remove the flash from the clinical set-up and simply switch to using the alternative systems as the camera set-up is totally different. Consideration should be given to purchasing a second camera and lens or just a body and using the lens from the clinical kit. A hybrid set up as **Figure 42** could be considered as a one camera system.

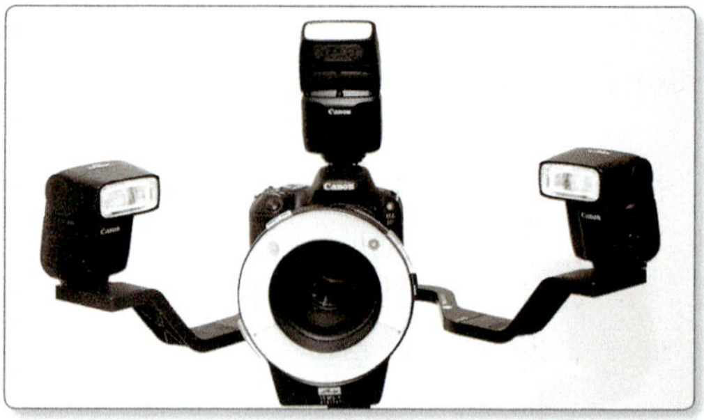

Figure 42 Combination bracket and lens mounted flash systems.

8 Comparison of lighting systems for faces

Facial photography using basic equipment

This section will be limited to recording faces as part of a clinical record.

The dental chair is convenient, but thought must be given to the background. The simple expedient of placing a suitably coloured card behind the patient can transform an image taken in the chair (**Figures 1a** and **b**).

Red eye

A frequent problem with on or near axis illumination of faces is that of "Red Eye". When the subject looks straight at the lens, light from the flash can be reflected directly back from the retina to the camera. Most if not all software programmes can deal easily with this phenomenon.

While it is possible to set up camera flash systems to avoid "Red Eye", this function should be disabled as it will trigger a pre-flash every time the flash is used (**Figures 2a** and **b**).

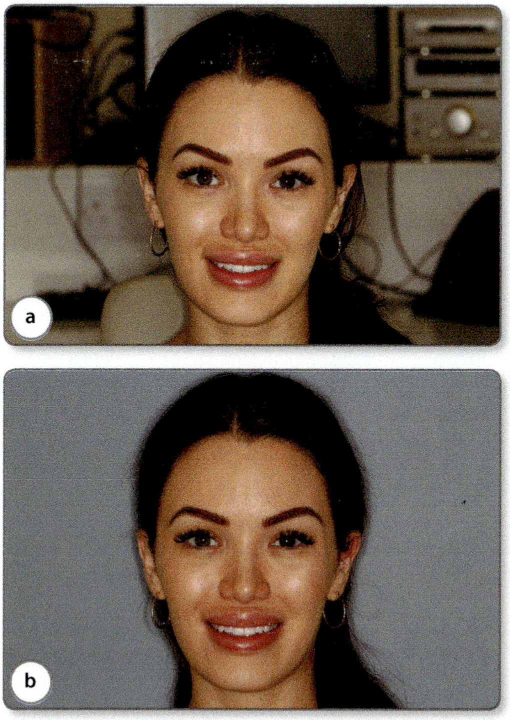

Figure 1 (a) Image taken in dental chair, (b) A1 card behind patient's head.
(*Courtesy:* Dr Mahul Patel)

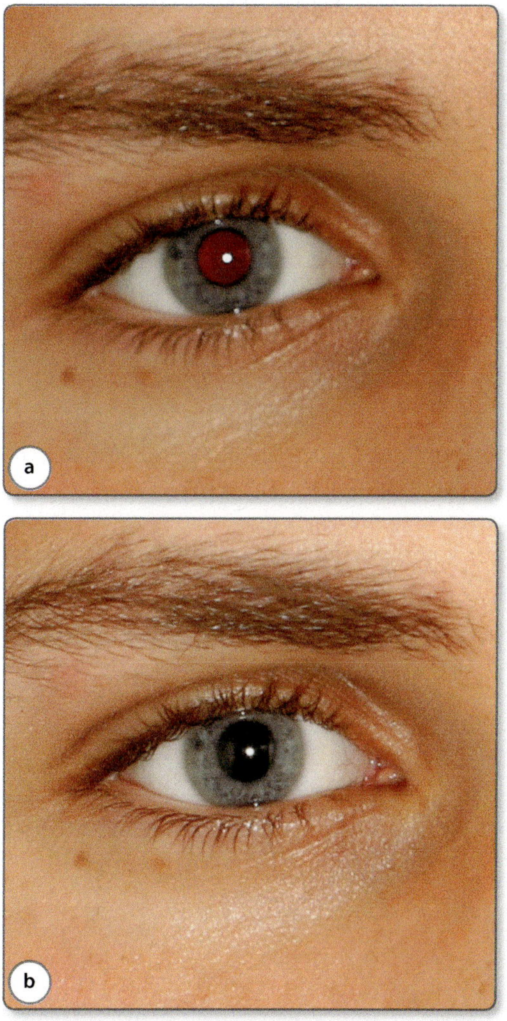

Figure 2 (a) Red eye Canon MR EX II Flash, (b) Red eye corrected.

Ideally both the operator and patient should be seated as this facilitates having the camera at the same height at the patient's head.

Backgrounds

Any direct lighting will produce shadows except on black velvet. The closer the subject to the background, the less obtrusive the shadow, also the closer the flash to the lens, the less the shadow (**Figures 3a** to **c**).

Other background colours may reduce the impact of the shadows but will not eliminate them (**Figures 4a** and **b**).

Black is common choice that can almost eliminate shadows but can also cause minor exposure problems. Black card, being slightly reflective as shown here, does not always come out as a true black. In this example against a black card, the automatic flash-metering has not coped with the virtually nonreflective background and overexposed the face (**Figure 5**).

Similarly, a very reflective white background can have the opposite effect and under expose the face (**Figure 6**). This problem can be minimised by presetting the camera metering system to "Spot" or "Centre-Weighted Average". One can of course select a mid range colour for the background (**Figures 7a** and **b**).

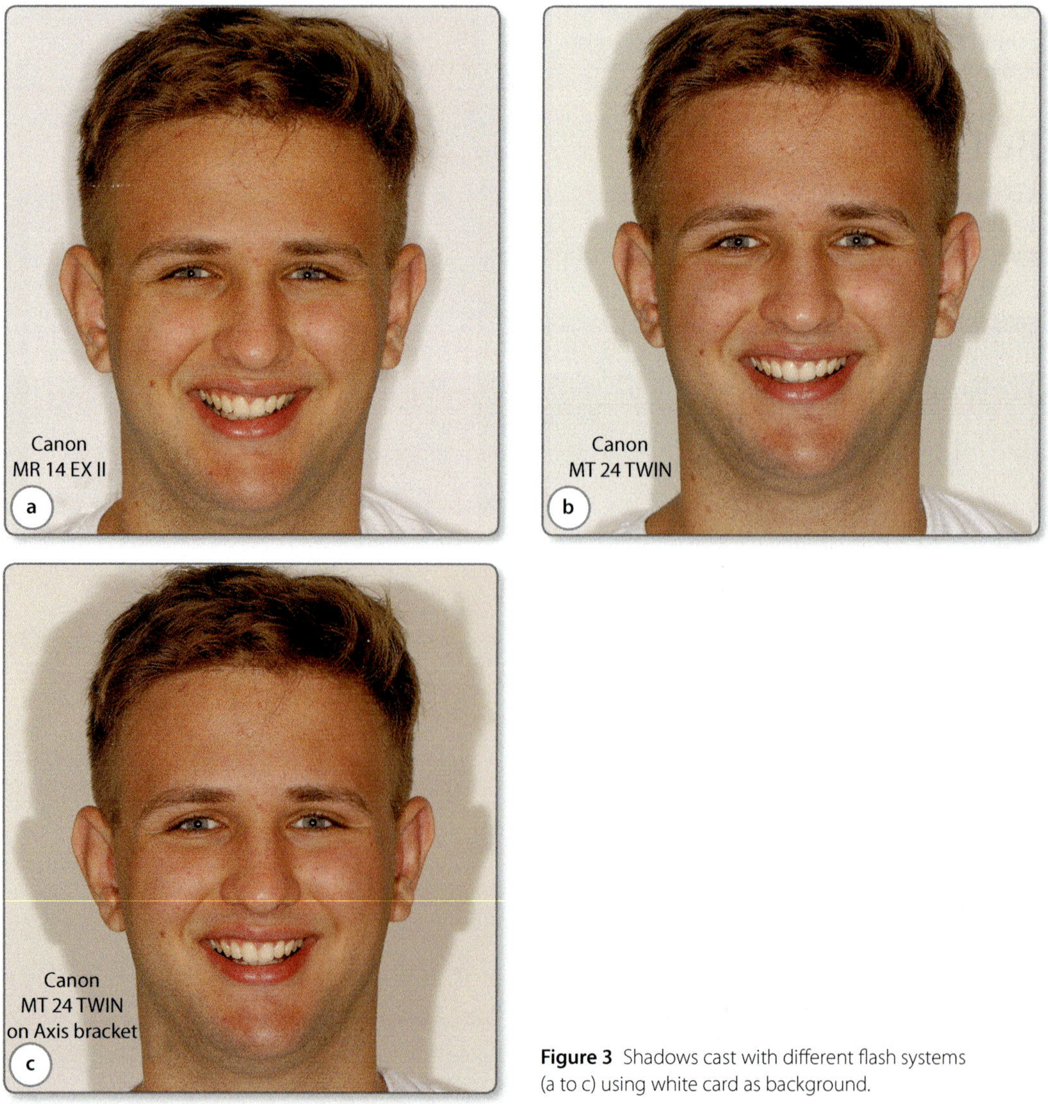

Figure 3 Shadows cast with different flash systems (a to c) using white card as background.

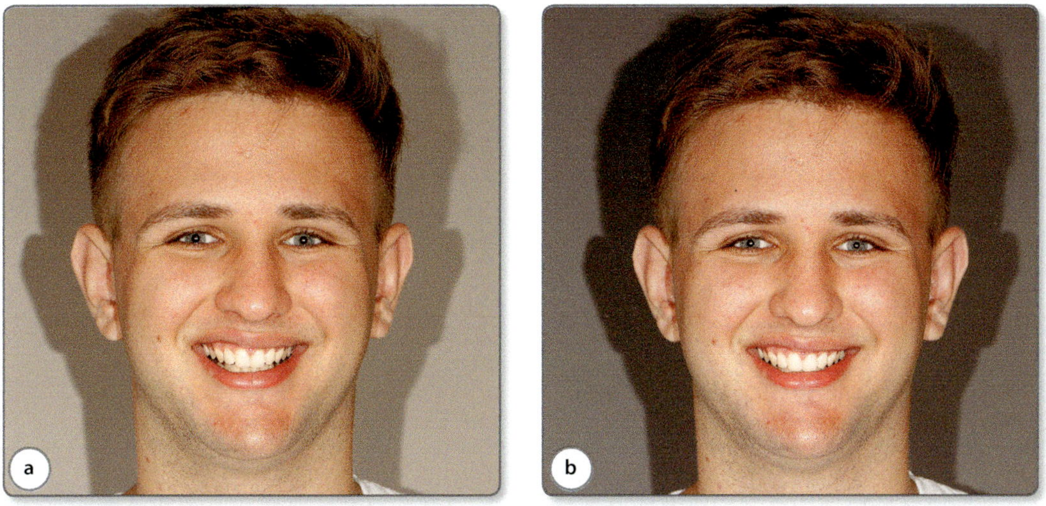

Figure 4 MT 24 Twin Flash with light and mid grey backgrounds (a and b).

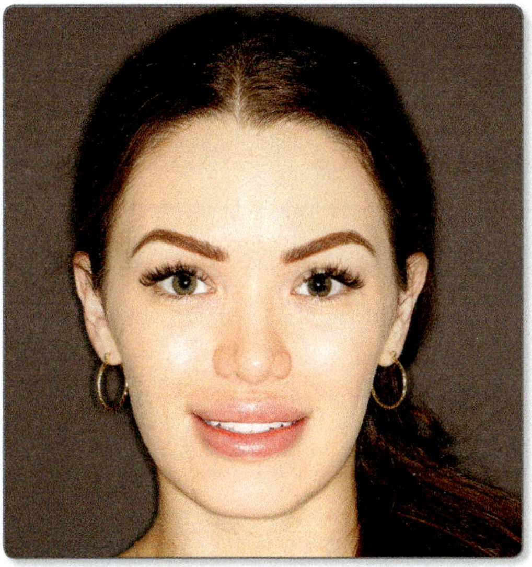

Figure 5 Black card background.
(*Courtesy*: Dr Mahul Patel)

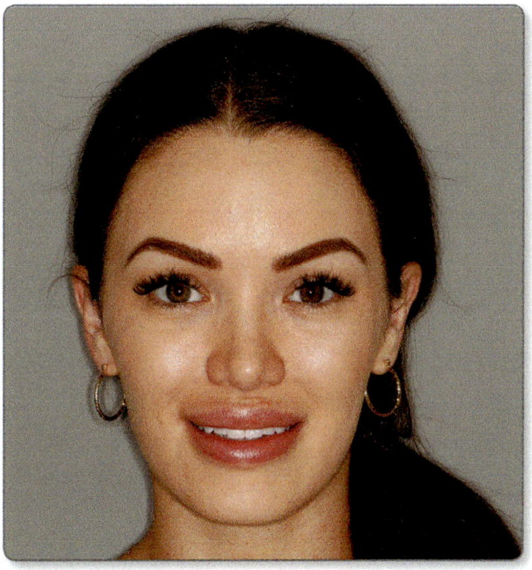

Figure 6 White card background.
(*Courtesy*: Dr Mahul Patel)

For a true black background, the author suggests black velvet which will virtually eliminate all shadows (**Figure 8**), but is not flattering to patients with black hair.

Shadows

Virtually all flash systems utilise two tubes and these are invariably placed at the 9 o' clock and 3 o'clock positions (**Figure 9a**).

For profile views by only using the flash on the side of the nose, the shadow can be limited to behind the head (**Figure 9b**).

There are light-emitting diode (LED) illuminated backgrounds available which tend to be very expensive. A cheap option is to purchase a 600 × 600 mm LED ceiling panel for under £50.00. They are very thin, framed and easily hung on a wall (**Figures 10** and **11**).

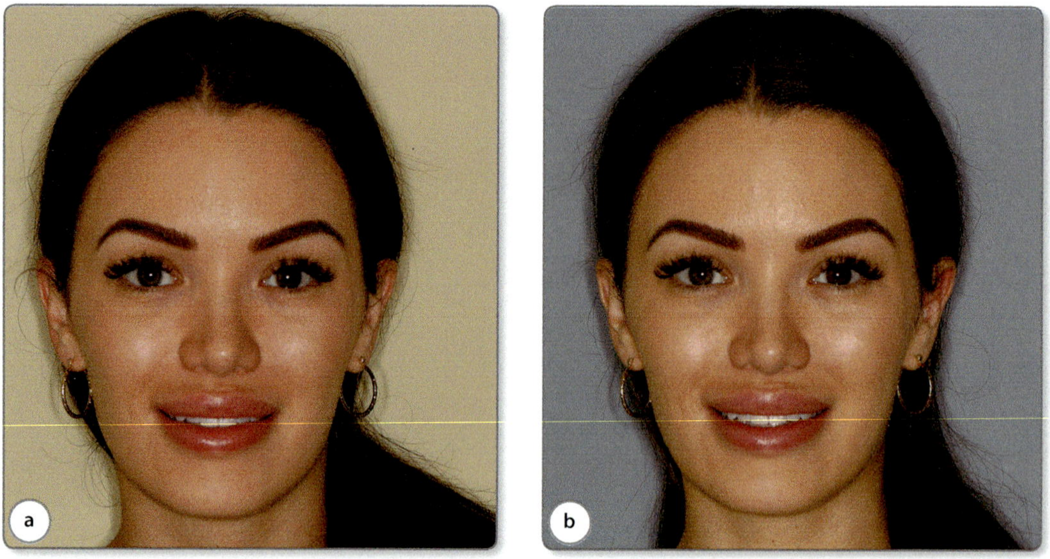

Figures 7a and b Images using pastel shades for background. (*Courtesy:* Dr Mahul Patel)

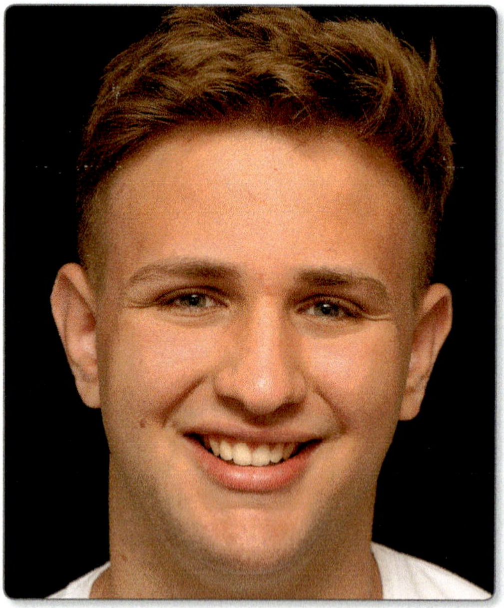

Figure 8 True black background using velvet.

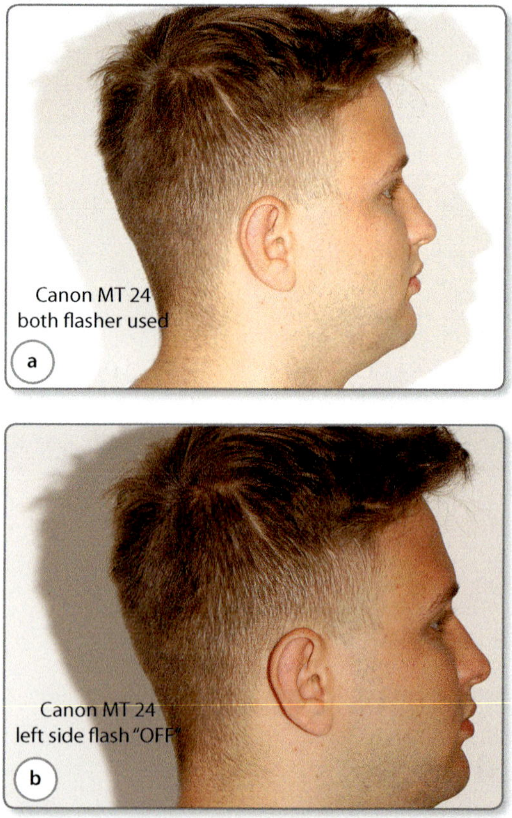

Figures 9 (a) Canon MT 24 – both flashes used, (b) Canon MT 24 – left side flash off.

Figure 10 Typical 600 × 600 mm light panel.

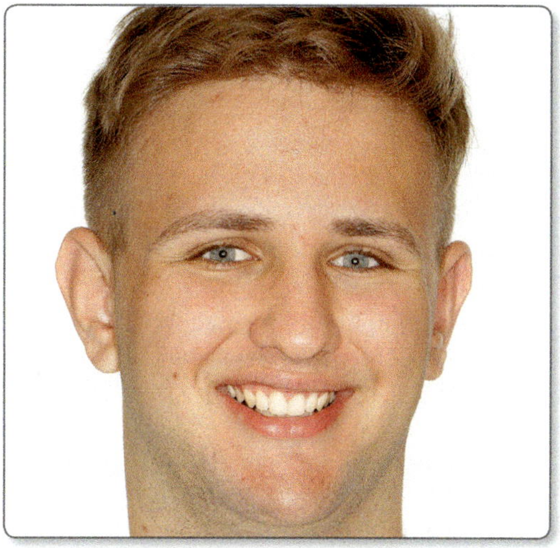

Figure 11 Image taken against light panel.

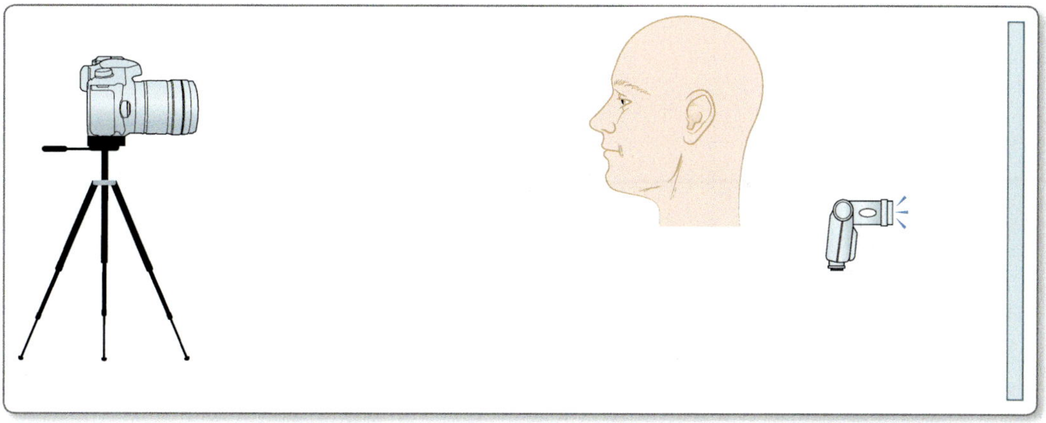

Figure 12 Slave flash unit.

Photographic images of patients today are often used far more widely than being restricted to the clinical records and it is mandatory that appropriate consent has been obtained for every intended source. Additionally, with the interest in facial aesthetics, the following might be considered.

Perhaps a caveat could be introduced at this point when considering "Before/After" photography.

> *"The main thing is to have the pictures as similar as possible—same background, same lighting, same angle, same hairstyle, same make up if any...etc. So that the only difference showing—hopefully—is the dramatic result of the aesthetic treatment."*
>
> **—Amanda Cameron**
> **Editor, Aesthetics Journal**

Slave flash

One very simple way to eliminate shadows from the subject is to place an additional "slave" flash unit, out of sight, between the subject and the background (**Figure 12**).

Figures 13a to **c** were taken using the Canon MR EX II "ring," MT 24 Twin Flash, and EL 100 Flash units on an axis bracket against a white wall showing typical shadows.

Figure 14 shows how by placing a slave flash behind the subject the shadow is eliminated and the background colour is improved.

Slave flash units are available in different formats.

There are simple purpose built "slave flash" units with built in optical receivers such as the Polaroid (**Figure 15**). These are triggered by the main flash on the camera.

In the absence of a purpose built slave flash an existing flash unit can be triggered by seating it in an optical receiver as shown in **Figure 16**.

A third option is a flash gun with a "slave" function such as the Kenro KFL 101 (**Figure 17**).

However, there can be problems, in principle the function is simple, an optical receiver in the slave system responds to the source flash and triggers the slave unit instantaneously. In practice, with current systems for digital cameras, it is not that simple. Referring to through-the-lens (TTL) metering in Chapter 1 the flash cycle of current units for digital photography incorporates a pilot or preflash followed almost immediately by the actual exposure flash. The author has found that the pilot flash triggers the slave units prematurely and accurate exposure or shadow elimination fails. It is possible, however, to set up many current systems to be used as slave units. The Kenro Speedflash KFL 101, for

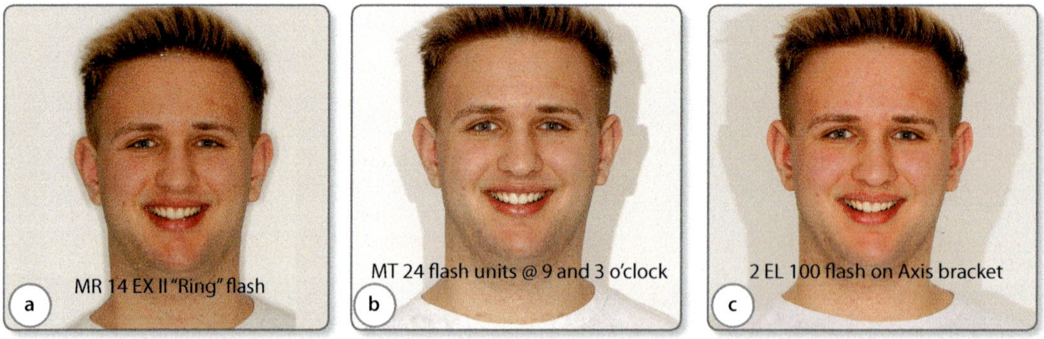

Figures 13a to c Images against white background.

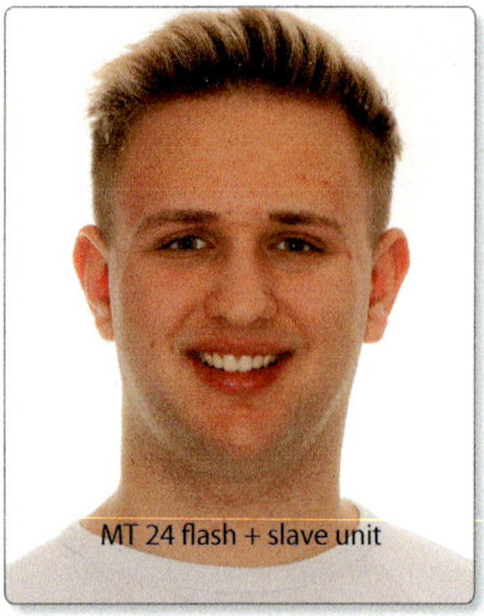

Figure 14 MT 24 Twin Flash and slave unit behind the subject.

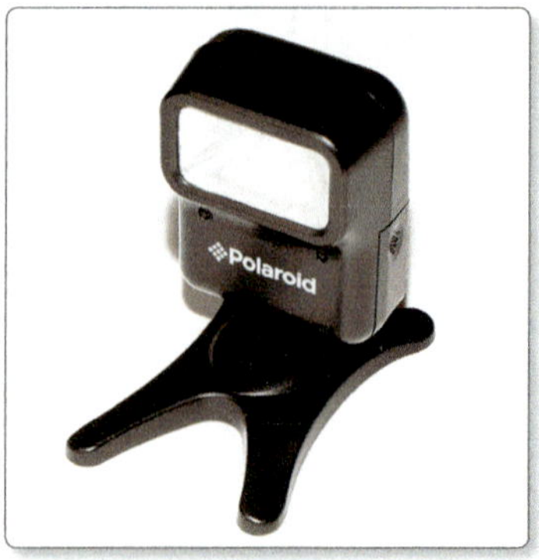

Figure 15 Polaroid slave flash.

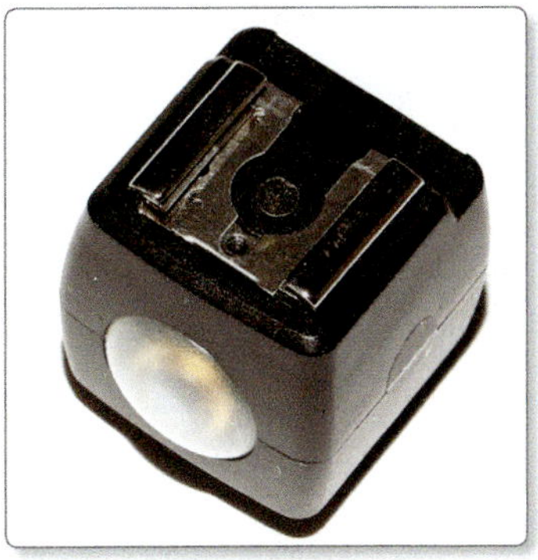

Figure 16 Optical hot shoe receiver.

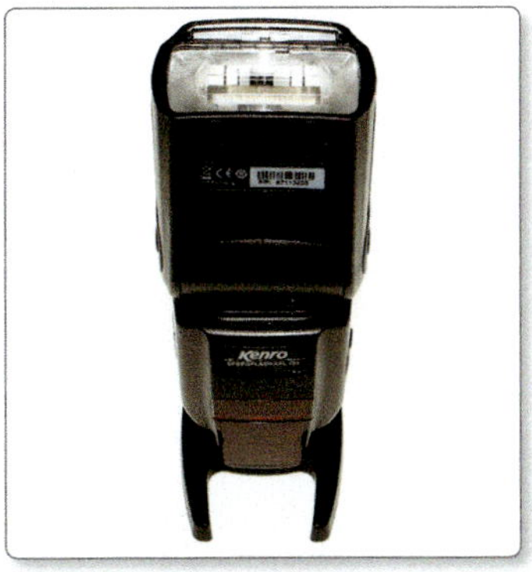

Figure 17 Kenro KFL 101 with master/slave facility.

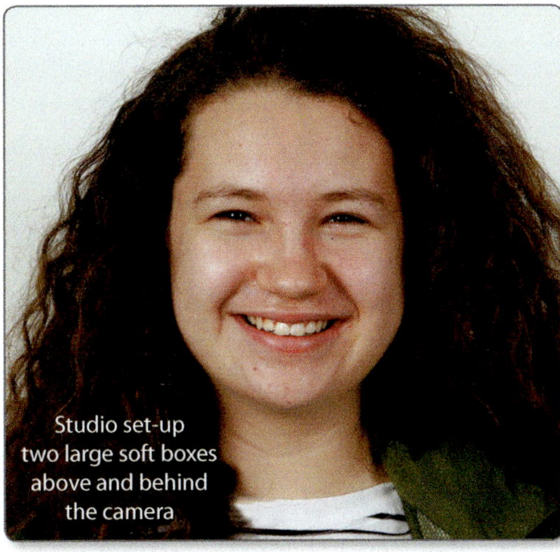

Figure 18 Image using studio flash (Knight Dental Design).

example in **Figure 17**, can be programmed to be triggered by specific "commander" flashes and ignore the latter's preflash. Nikon and Canon flash systems also offer these facilities on latest models.

Most systems now rely on radio wireless transmission to trigger slave flashes, the advantage being that a direct line of sight between master and slave is not required.

All the above suggestions are designed just to fire the slave flash to illuminate the background and independent of the TTL control of the flash illuminating the subject.

Facial photography

If you have a camera set up with a "Ring Flash", the most expedient way of capturing a facial shot is to make any necessary setting change to the camera (usually a change from f22 to f8) and use it. Any of the following options, will require "dismantling" of the clinical set up or setting up a separate dedicated "portrait" kit. Remember the position of the light source/s will influence both the background shadows and the shadows produced by facial features, nose, ears and chin for example.

This facial image (**Figure 18**) was taken in a studio courtesy Knight Dental Design Laboratory against a white wall. Note the catch lights in the eyes indicating the double light source which comprised two large soft boxes placed above and behind the camera.

Flash systems for faces

Figures 19 to **36** were taken with various accessories against a white background.

The Canon 470EX-AI (**Figure 37**) incorporates a motorised flash head and is programmed to select a good flash position for different shooting situations. **Figures 37a** and **b** show how incorporating more of the subject and introducing a pose, a "Mug Shot" can very easily become a portrait.

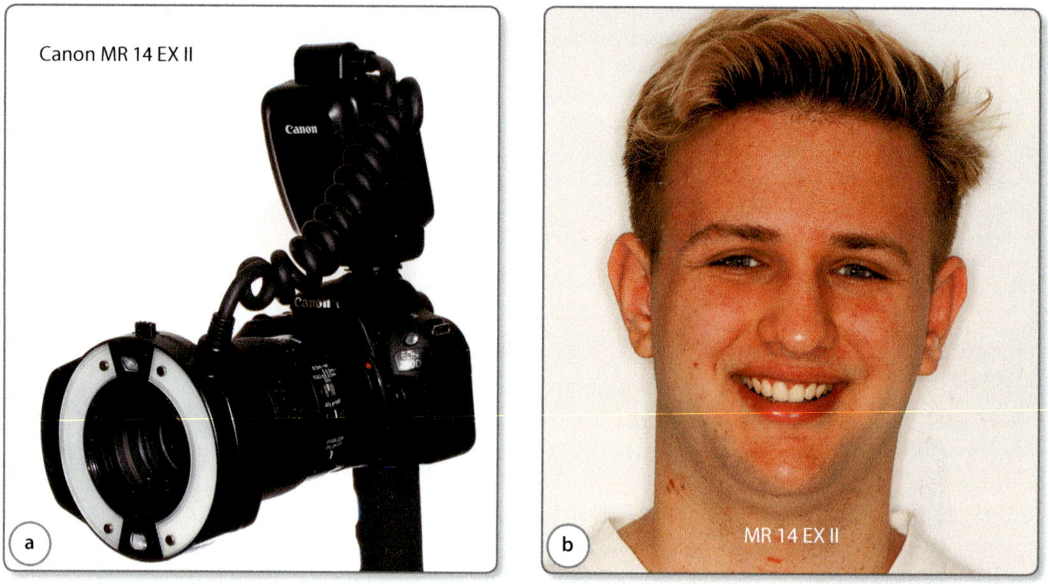

Figure 19 (a) Canon MR 14 EX II; (b) Image taken with standard clinical flash.

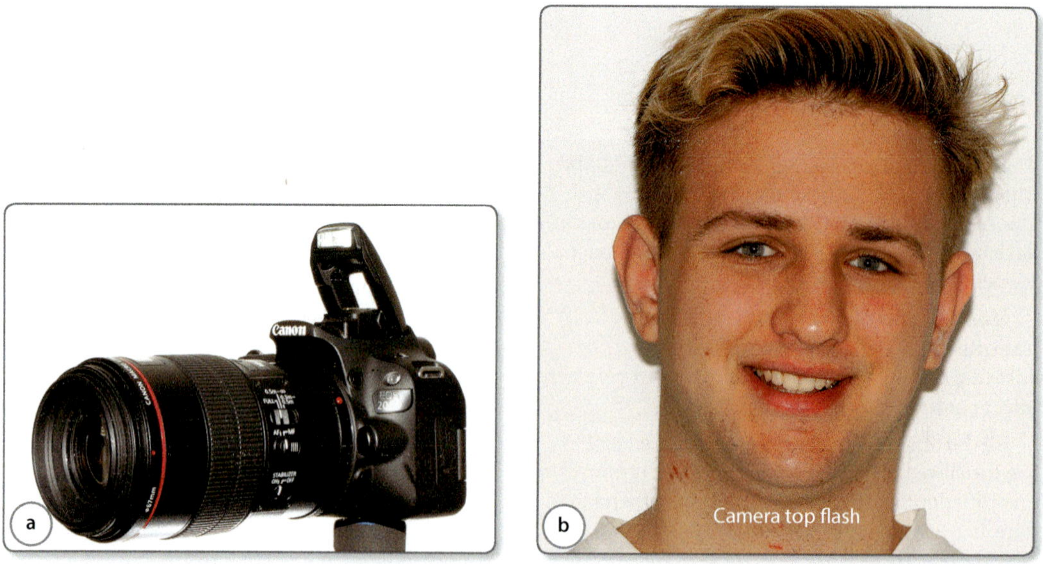

Figure 20 (a) Canon built in flash; (b) Image taken using camera's built in flash.

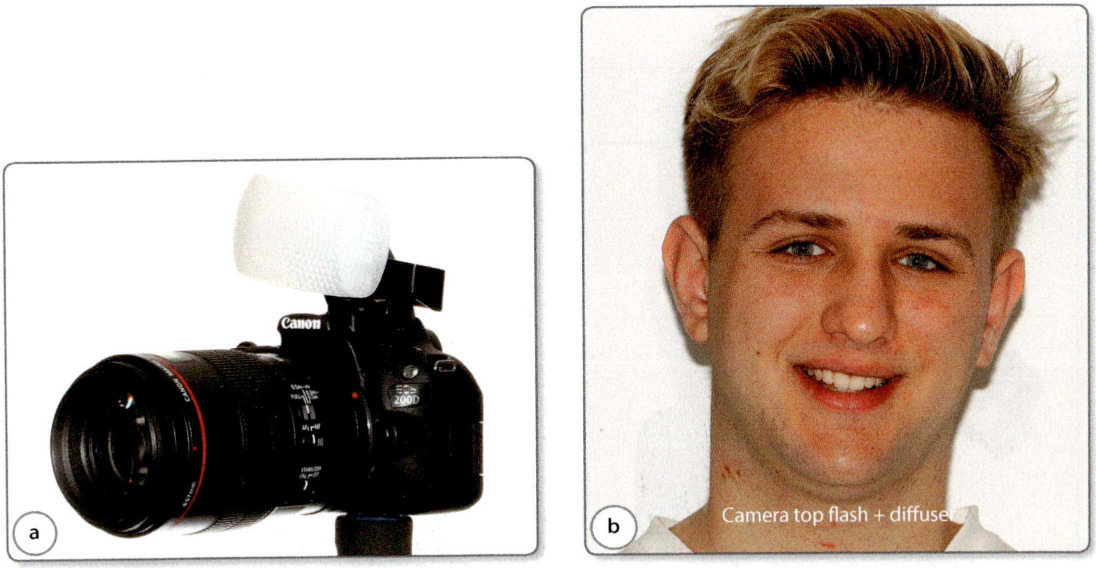

Figure 21 (a) Canon built in flash diffused; (b) Image taken with diffuser attached to camera's flash (note colour cast).

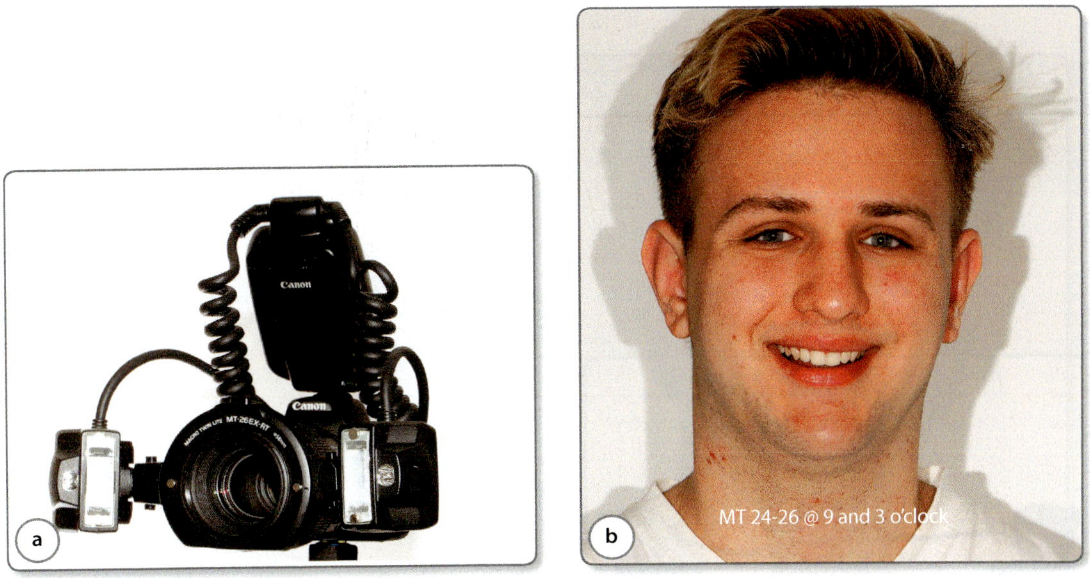

Figure 22 (a) Canon MT 24/26 at 9 and 3 o'clock; (b) Image taken with MT 24 Flash.

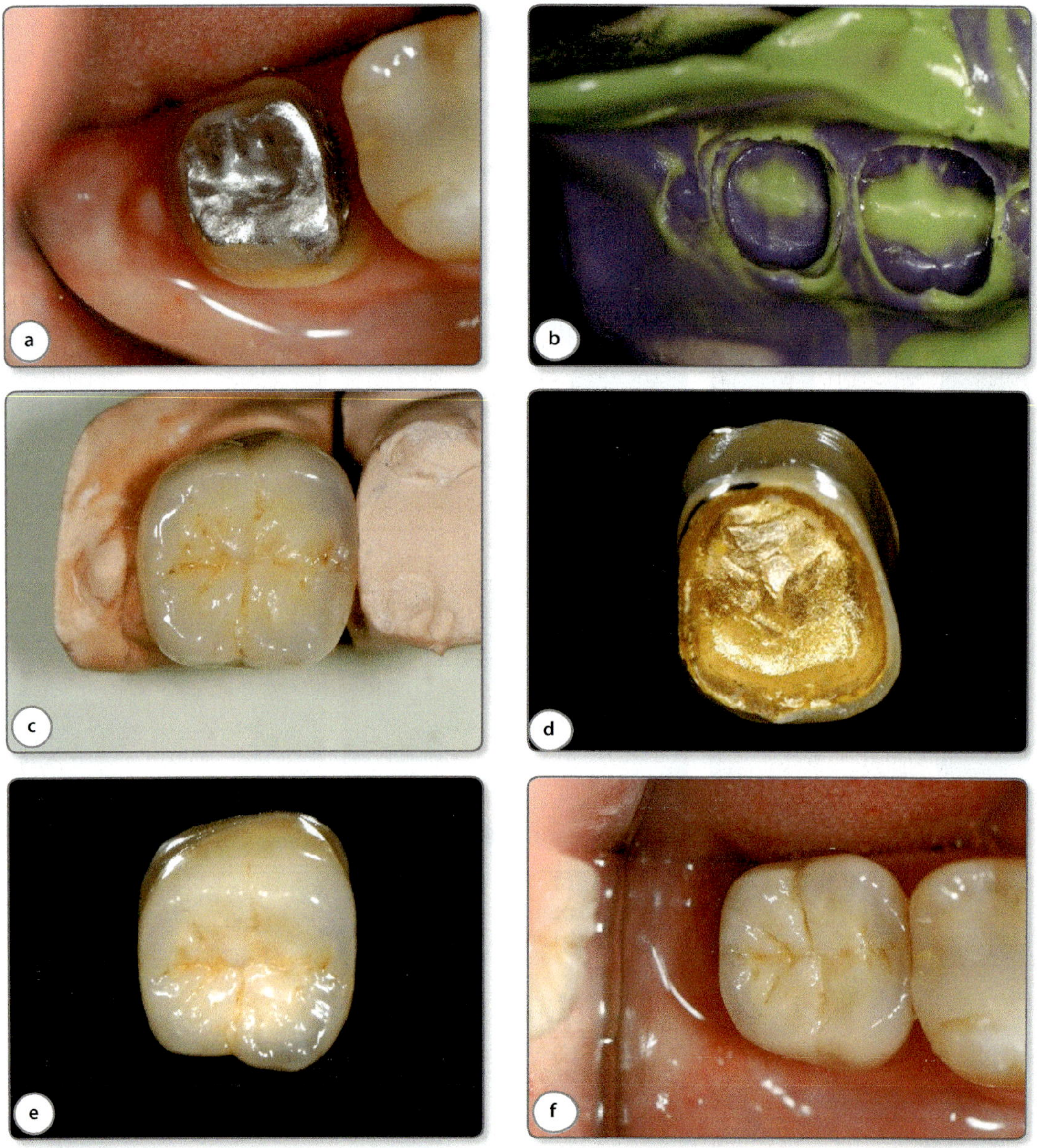

Figures 21a to f Series of images from preparation to final fit.
(*Courtesy*: Dr Anil Shrestha)

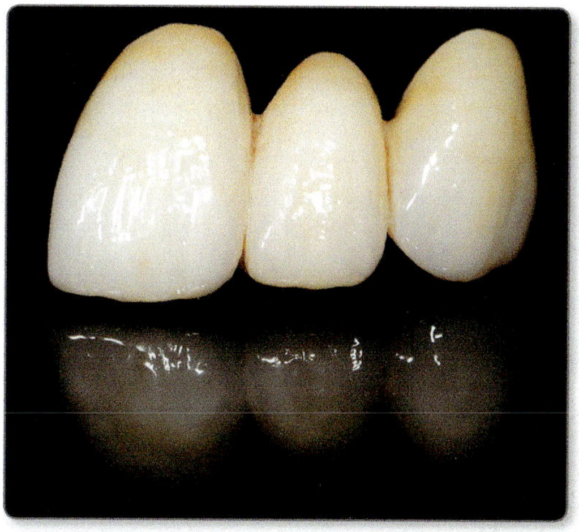

Figure 22 Black acrylic.

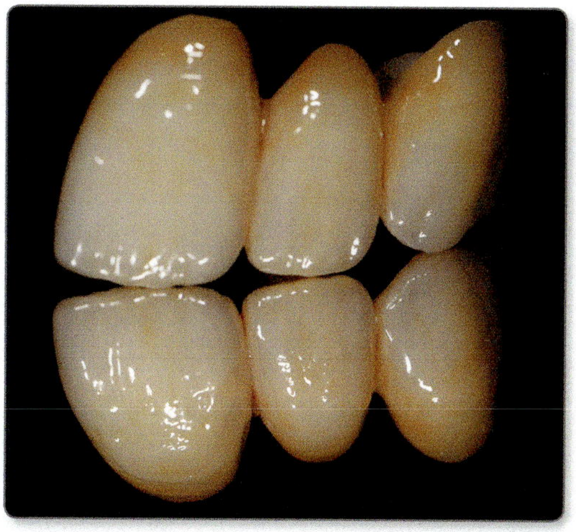

Figure 23 Ultrabright mirror.

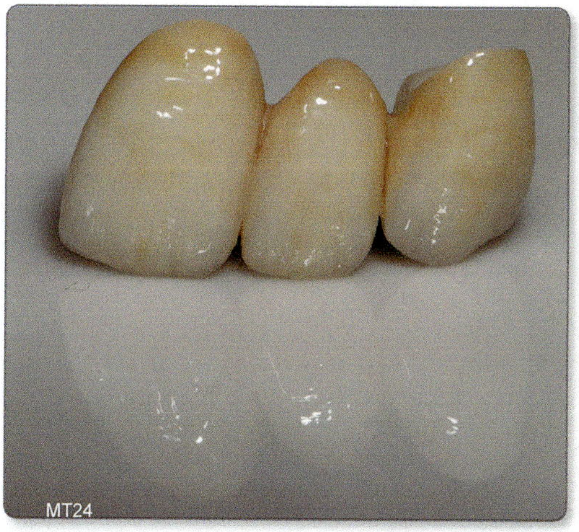

Figure 24 White acrylic.

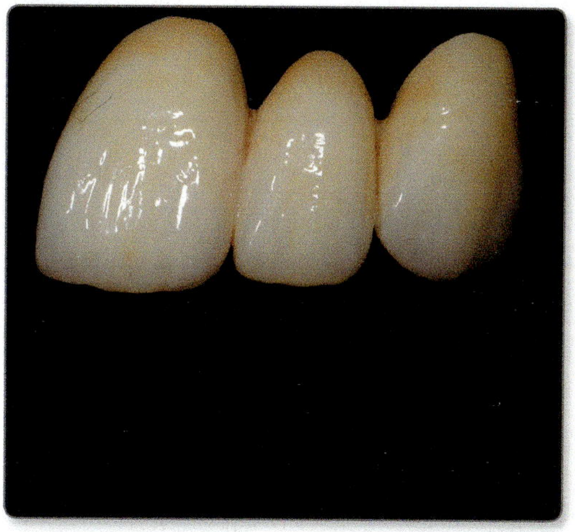

Figure 25 Black velvet.
(*Courtesy:* Bryan Matthews. Images by Dr P Gordon)

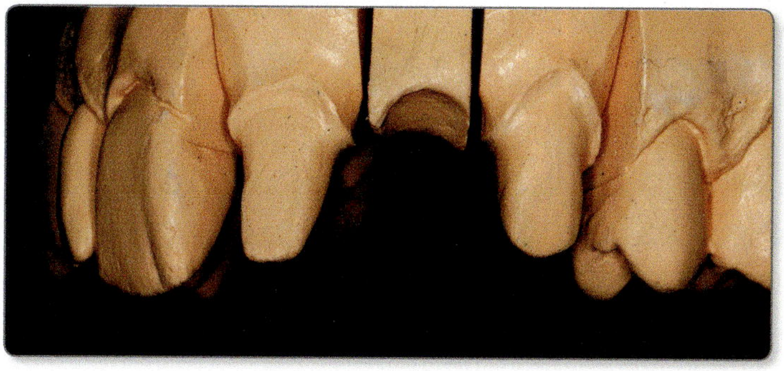

Figure 26 Stone model.

Specific Postgraduate requirements

College of medicine and dentistry

The College of Medicine and Dentistry formerly the BPP University require the following series of images for their Implant Course as illustrated by **Figures 33** to **35**. and would no doubt be similar to those required for restorative courses generally. In addition to the standard views as shown in **Figures 4**, **6**, **8**, and **9**, images of lips at rest and smiling are required (see **Figures 33** and **34**).

Study models in these circumstances need to be photographed on semi-adjustable articulators together with occlusal views removed from the articulators (see **Figure 35**).

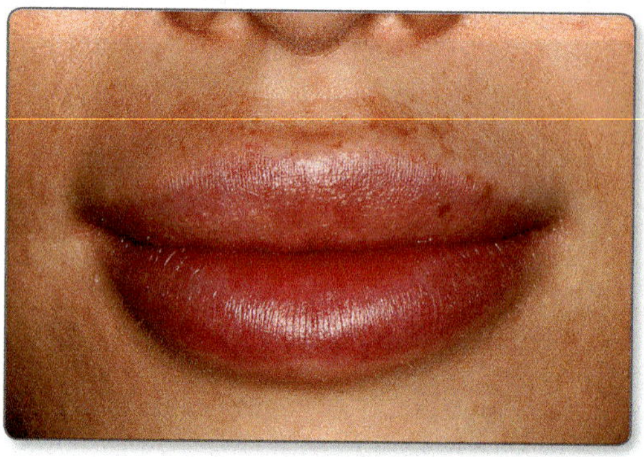

Figure 33 Lips together

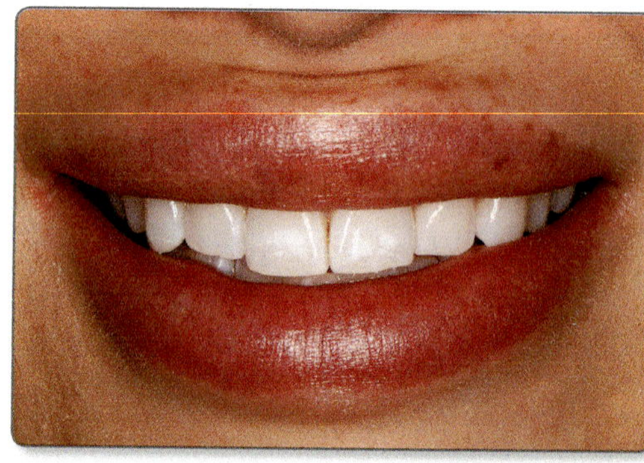

Figure 34 Lips apart

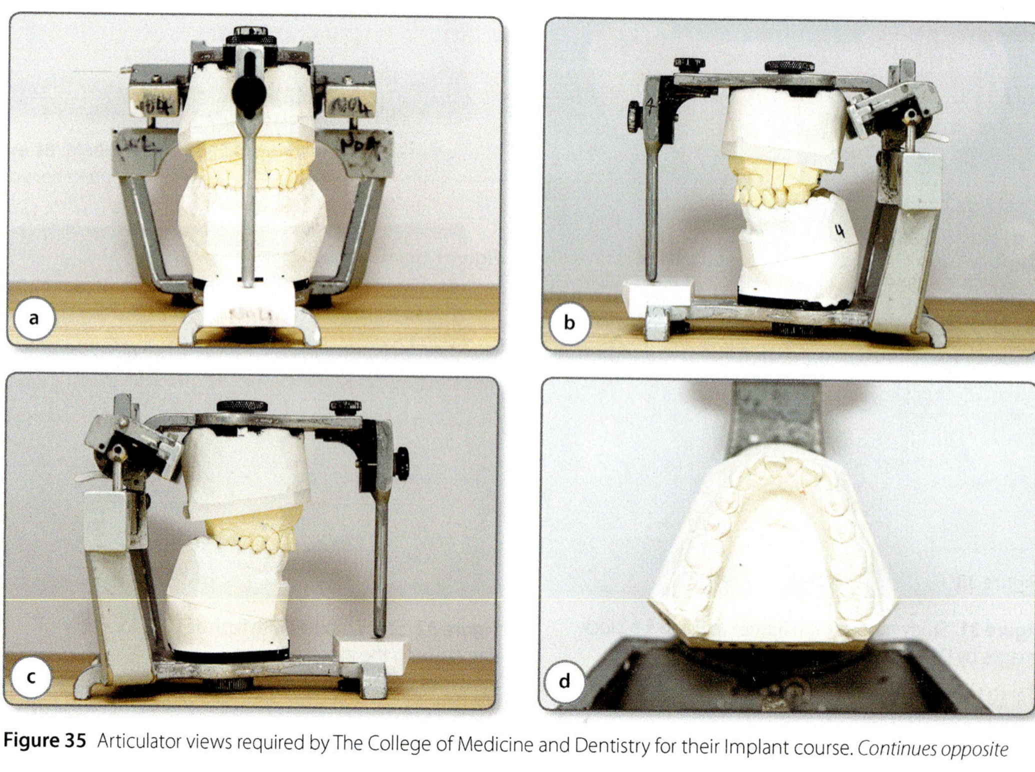

Figure 35 Articulator views required by The College of Medicine and Dentistry for their Implant course. *Continues opposite*

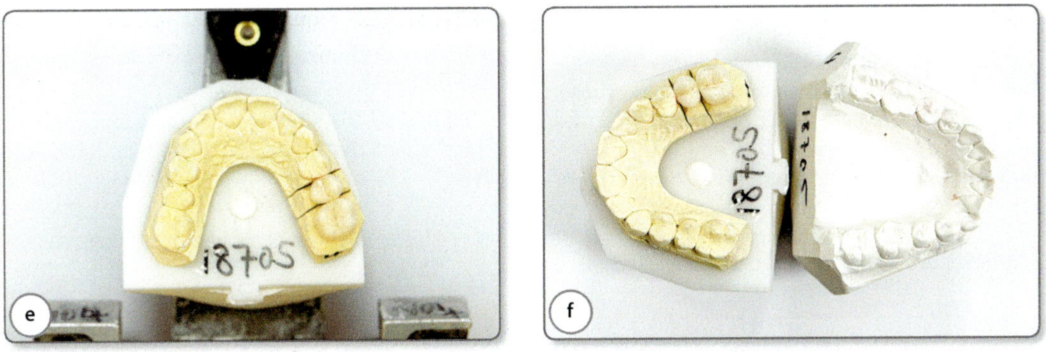

Figure 35 *Continued.*

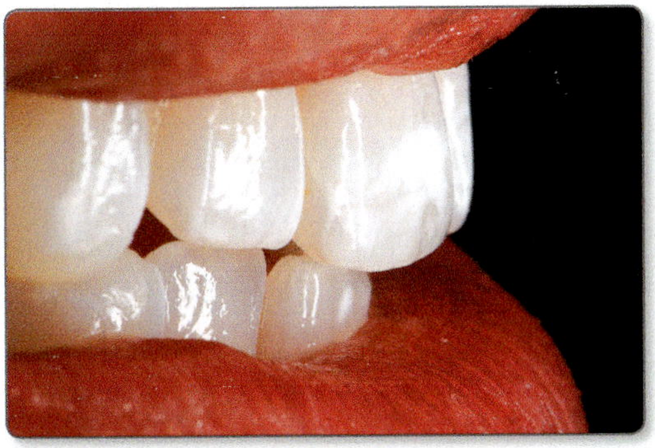

Figure 36 Ring flash on camera.
(*Courtesy:* Dr Mahut Patel)

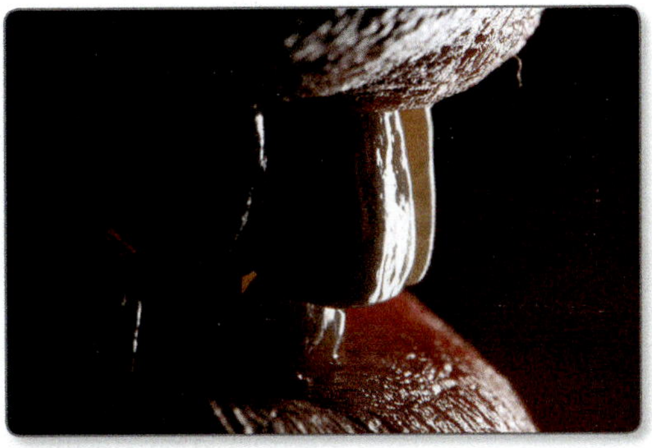

Figure 37 Ring flash held off camera.
(*Courtesy:* Dr Mahut Patel)

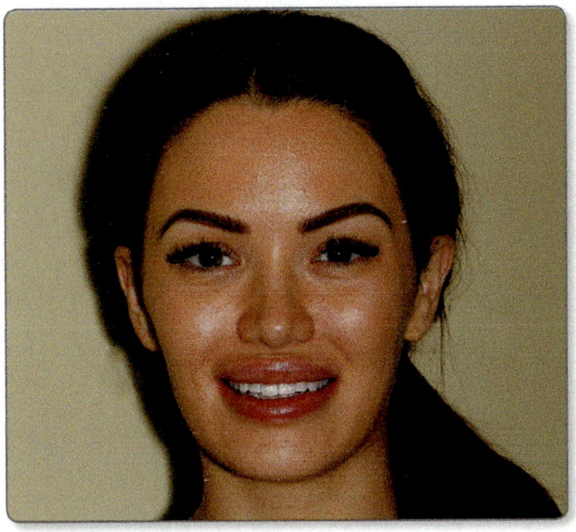

Figure 38 Ring flash on camera.
(*Courtesy:* Dr Mahut Patel)

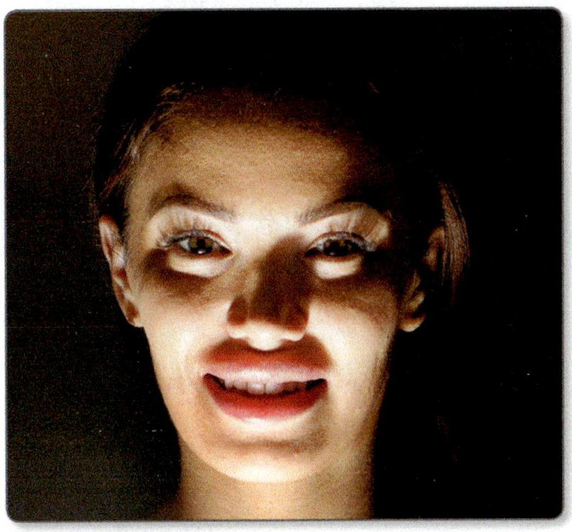

Figure 39 Ring flash to one side off camera.
(*Courtesy:* Dr Mahut Patel)

Non-clinical images

Eye catching images can be easily achieved by taking the flash head off the camera and experimenting. **Figures 36** to **39** were taken by Dr Mahul Patel. For greater versatility flash units etc .Single flash units can be used “off camera” and maintaining automatic metering by using an appropriate extension cable (see **Figure 40**).

Creative filters

The mirrorless Canon M50 and the DSLR's 200D and 250D all incorporate "creative" filters. These effects can be created on existing images which are then saved as separate files on the memory card and the original is maintained. Seven filters are available and on the DSLR's there is a choice of degrees of change. The following images show three of the effects.

Figures 41 to **43**, show the "grainy black and white" effect, the 'fish eye' view and the "art bold effect".

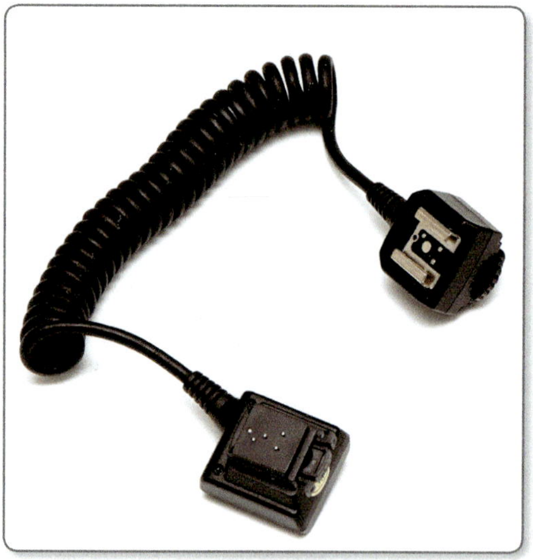

Figure 40 Through-the-Lens (TTL) extension cord.

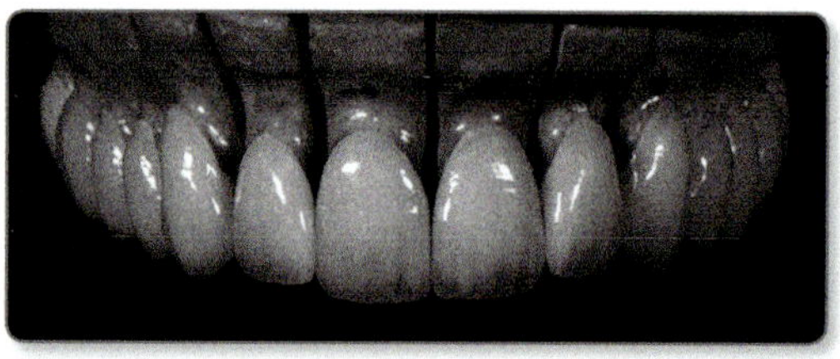

Figure 41 Black & white grainy effect.

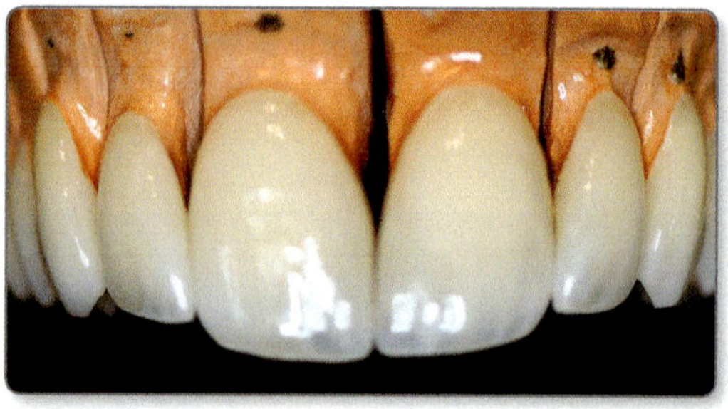

Figure 42 Fish eye effect.

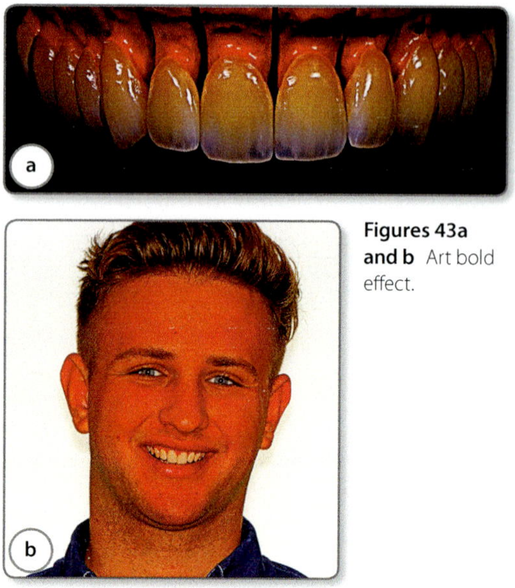

Figures 43a and b Art bold effect.

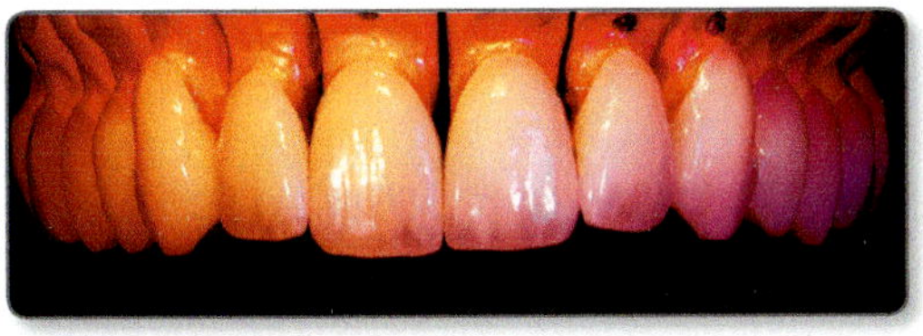

Figure 44 Photography with Adaptalux lighting system.

Adaptalux

Figure 44, used on the cover, was shot using the Adaptalux lighting system. Currently the LED light source is provided by flexible arms with detachable white or coloured shades (**Figure 45**). The light output is relatively low so that mounting the camera on a tripod is essential. It is understood that a flash source is currently being developed which should facilitate cameras being handheld.

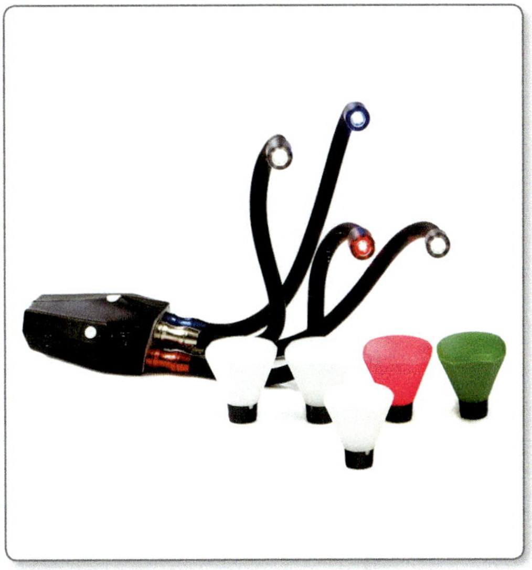

Figure 45 Colour LED lights for photography.

Index

Note: Page numbers in **bold** or *italic* refer to tables or figures, respectively.